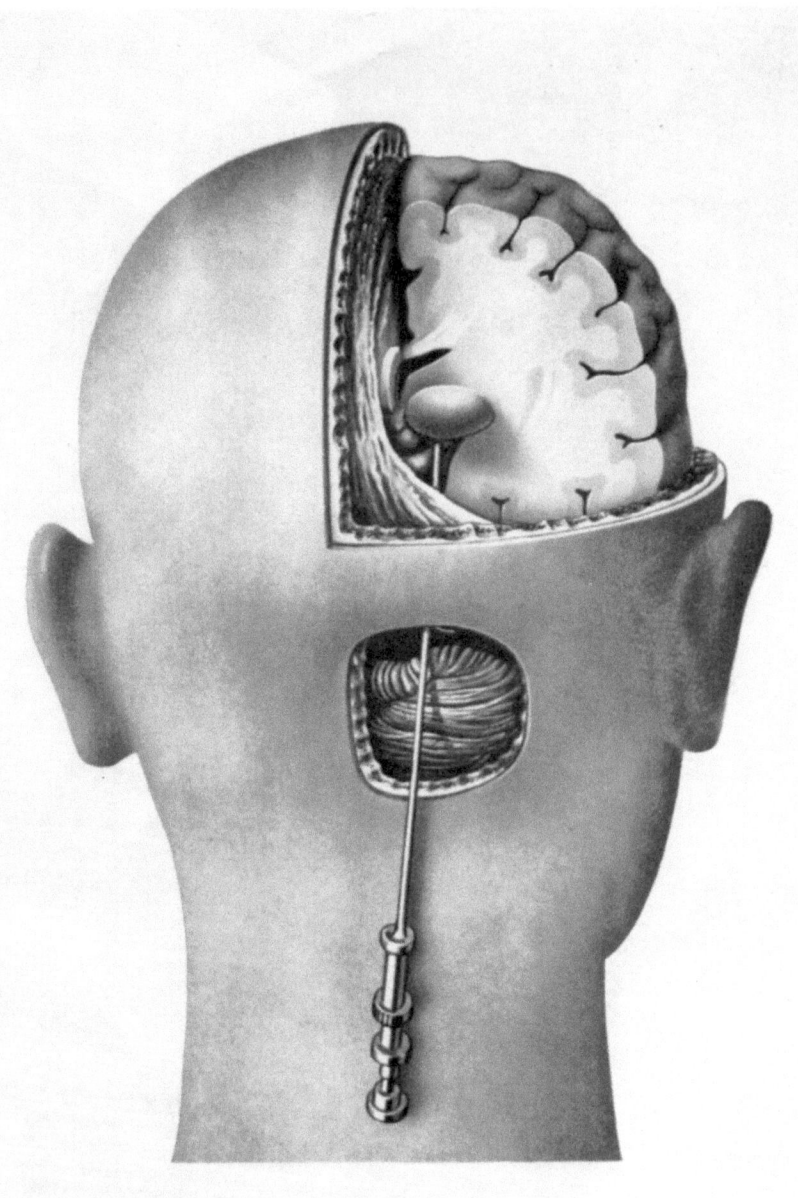

ACTA NEUROCHIRURGICA / SUPPLEMENTUM XVIII

Open
Mesencephalotomy and Thalamotomy
for Intractable Pain

By

Bohuslav Zapletal, M. D.

Associate Professor of Neurological Surgery
Palacký University School of Medicine and Hospital
Olomouc, Czechoslovakia

With 29 Figures

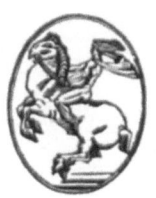

1969

SPRINGER-VERLAG / WIEN · NEW YORK

ISBN-13: 978-3-7091-8240-6   e-ISBN-13: 978-3-7091-8238-3
DOI: 10.1007/978-3-7091-8238-3

Titel Nr. 9251

To my teacher
Professor Vladislav Rapant, M. D., Dr. Sc.
to whom modern surgery in Czechoslovakia
is greatly indebted

Acknowledgements

I am much indebted to Mr. F. MIKULA, M. D., Professor of Neurology and to Mr. V. VÁŇA, M. D., Olomouc, Czechoslovakia, for their continuous enthusiastic cooperation and their participation in the care and study of the patients operated on for intractable pain, to Mr. F. KAPITAN, for his valuable assistance in providing the technical illustrations, and to Mr. F. LIPPER for the skilful construction of the loop-scalpel. In the same way I wish to thank Mrs. N. WOOD and Mr. J. V. BLUMBERG, M. D., who were so kind as to translate the monograph from the Czech original.

Olomouc, December 1968

B. Zapletal

Contents

I. Introduction

Severe, protracted pain defying control is being seen with increasing frequency as a symptom of chronic disease. It accompanies many, mostly serious, disorders in various organs and parts of the human body, making the sufferer's life increasingly intolerable. It no longer fulfills its mission of warning signal of disease present, protecting health, but on the contrary arises as an important factor in systematically reducing and preparing the final collapse of the defensive forces of the body, both in the somatic and psychic spheres. It can surprise nobody that patients tormented and plagued by severe pain do not wish to live under conditions primarily caused by incurable disease, and are looking forward longingly to their release by death, if no help is forthcoming. Attempts to control such pain are, therefore entirely justified, necessary and logical.

The treatment of intractable pain is without exception symptomatic in character. Efforts to control it by drugs are, even at present and despite the striking progress in pharmacology, unsatisfactory and inadequate. So far we know of no drug capable of effectively and systematically alleviating such pain without concurrently interfering with the other sensitive-sensory components. In addition to the direct changes and disturbances of consciousness and personality, protracted conservative therapy results in addiction to narcotics. Only in cases of life expectancy limited to a short period, or those not suited for any type of surgery, have we to make do with conservative treatment. We decide in favour of radical therapy in all others, which at present mainly signifies an attack on the secondary pain pathway in spinal cord and brain stem.

The ascending spinal pathways, conducting painful and thermal stimuli are, however, not represented only by the well-defined, narrow and constant bundle of nerve fibres figuring in the illustrations of many textbooks up to the present. Afferent fibres extend over a wide area of the anterolateral quadrant of the cord and the medulla, becoming more and more diffuse, intermingled with other sensory pathways and forming a mono- and polysynaptic network with the reticular formation and many nuclei of the stem on the same and opposite sides in the regions of the pons, mesencephalon, thalamus and subthalamus. On the other hand, it was ascertained

that the pain fibres in the classical lateral spinothalamic tract are
arranged segmentally, throughout the entire pathway terminating
in the thalamus. Facts mentioned so far, as well as others, make
the study of problems concerning the radical treatment of intractable pain a highly interesting as well as exacting one.

Metastases are the most common cause of "surgical" pain. We
observe them with increasing frequency, mainly because we are
becoming increasingly, though slowly, more successful in prolonging
the life of these patients. Their increasing frequency is responsible
for the increasing experience of neurosurgeons with their treatment.
From results of such operations, the surgeon is able to draw most
important data on surgical technique, clinical and physiological
facts and so select the optimal site for intervention, again by experiences gained, thus enhancing the therapeutic effect. Important
progress in this field has been made especially in recent years.

Much more exacting and far less rewarding is the neurosurgeon's
task as regards suppression of so-called central pain. Its most common representative is thalamic and phantom pain. In such cases
pain "fixed" right up to the highest brain levels cannot be controlled
by operation limited to the long fibres of the spinothalamic tract.
More extensive operations must be tried out, as will be referred to
later, or a different conservative or perhaps combined therapy. So
far, however, central pain remains an unrewarding chapter to the
neurosurgeon, neurologist, or any other therapist for that matter.

There are many sites where the secondary pain pathway has been
transected in years past. The long drawn-out history of these operations points to the fact that surgeons had to advance gradually and
cautiously from the periphery to the centre, i.e. from the spinal
cord up to the region of the thalamus, impeded by lack of knowledge on structure-function, as well as by shortcomings of technical
equipment. It is not surprising, therefore, that from the first modest
operation for pain done by MARTIN on the spinal cord in the year
1911—upper thoracic cordotomy was the operation in question—
up to the time when the spinothalamic tract was first destroyed
at its termination in the thalamus, almost 40 years have elapsed.
An important role in this successful advance was played by stereotaxis.

This paper deals with problems of surgical treatment for intractable pain especially in these highest sectors of the secondary pain
pathway, in the mesencephalon, on the mesencephalothalamic
junction and thalamus. This was facilitated and simplified by the
elaboration of an infratentorial route of approach to both the above-
mentioned structures during the years 1954—1956. With the full

and active support of my teacher, director of the Surgical University Clinic in Olomouc, Professor V. RAPANT, this method of surgical intervention has been further developed and improved. It was used not only in surgery for pain, but also for some expansive lesions, for surgery of extrapyramidal disorders—nigrotomy and subthalamotomy—and finally for the investigation of the pineal gland in man—pinealectomy.

Starting in the year 1955, the writer has performed various operations for intractable pain on the midbrain, the junction of the mesencephalon and thalamus and in the thalamic region itself, on 51 patients. All these interventions were done by the open infratentorial technique of approach. This number is, of course, insufficient for drawing final conclusions and making decisions on the various types of interventions. However, this is the largest personal series of mesencephalotomies, mesencephalothalamotomies and thalamosubthalamotomies altogether. In conjunction with the experiences of other neurosurgeons performing mesencephalotomies by WALKER's open transtentorial route or stereotactically, or, as the case may be, thalamotomy with subthalamotomy by stereotaxis, it can contribute not only to the highly desirable improvement of clinical results, but may become an important contribution for further research and progress in the field of neurophysiology.

II. A History of Operations on the Mesencephalon and Thalamus

The period of most rapid progress of neurosurgery definitely belongs to the first third of this century thanks to HARVEY CUSHING (1869—1939) and others who devised those fundamental surgical techniques for a majority of the areas of the brain which are being used to the present day. However, as regards the mesencephalon and thalamus, conditions prevailing at that time could not be expected to provide the necessary basis for perfect and safe surgical interventions. Systematic research and the endeavour to penetrate to these regions were impeded by the lack of technical facilities as well as by gaps in knowledge respecting the anatomy and functional role of both structures. Sporadically performed interventions in man met as a rule with failure by seriously interfering either directly or indirectly with neighbouring or more distant cerebral structures and causing severe neurological deficits, thus discrediting the experiment or therapeutic intervention and directly endangering the patient's life. What is more, this first period of sporadic operations did not have the object of directly affecting the functions of either mesencephalon or thalamus. The history of direct incisions or punctures in the various areas of the brain stem or medulla with the object of interrupting certain groups of tracts or nuclei, is much more recent (SJÖQVIST, 1937) than operations for neoplastic, inflammatory or congenital diseases of these structures or their immediate neighbourhood.

The first to attempt the radical removal of an expansively growing lesion in this region, a tumour of the pineal gland, was probably the Englishman VICTOR HORSLEY (1857—1916). Details about this operation performed in the year 1910 are unfortunately not available. HORSLEY himself stated that he selected an infratentorial approach. However, the operation met with so many complications that he envisaged further advances in this line of surgery only by using the supratentorial route. Despite this, OPPENHEIM and KRAUSE reported in 1913 the case of a patient in whom they successfully removed a tumour of the pineal gland by the infratentorial route, from an occipitosuboccipital craniotomy and with elevation of the tentorium. However, the second operation done by KRAUSE in 1926 for the same condition proved a failure.

NASSETTI in 1913 chose a very radical approach consisting of the resection of the sagittal sinus, falx and straight sinus followed by transection of the posterior part of the corpus callosum. However, this route which carried great risks was never used again. BRUNNER in the same year used an approach by occipital craniotomy, retracting the occipital lobe upward and transecting the corpus callosum. TANDLER and RANZI in 1920 modified this operation of BRUNNER by transecting the tentorium alongside the straight sinus. PUUSEPP in 1914 performed an occipital paramedian craniotomy, opened the dura over the right occipital lobe, ligated the right transverse sinus and transected the tentorium alongside the straight sinus on the right. After this he evacuated the liquid contents of the cystic growth leaving the tumour itself of necessity behind. The patient died on the third postoperative day. In 1921 DANDY recommended a transcallosal approach from a large parietooccipital craniotomy for operations in the region of the posterior portion of the third ventricle and pineal gland, after first testing this surgical technique by performing pinealectomy in dogs. FÖRSTER in 1928 tried the approach by occipital craniotomy, with simple retraction of the occipital lobe away from the tentorium and falx cerebri.

VAN WAGENEN in 1931 exploited the internal hydrocephalus accompanying expansively growing lesions in the region of the third ventricle for facilitating his approach to the pineal region through the dilated lateral ventricle. HORRAX in 1937 recommended a two stage procedure: during the first stage he resected the occipital part of the parietal lobe up to the splenium corporis callosi. The growth is removed during the second stage. BAGGENSTOSS and LOVE in 1939 also recommended a two-stage operation: part of the growth was removed during stage one by the transcallosal route, extirpation was completed during the second stage using an suboccipital craniotomy.

Results achieved by all the operations so far described were, however, never wholly satisfactory due to the difficult approach to growths in the region of the posterior part of the third ventricle and pineal gland, as well as on account of the very serious functional disorders associated with tumours in this locality. For the reasons mentioned many neurosurgeons up the present day prefer either TORKILDSEN's drainage operation, or simple subtemporal decompression and X-ray therapy, as recommended in 1942 by HORRAX and DANIELSEN, for the treatment of expansive lesions affecting this region.

The first surgeon who destroyed part of the mesencephalon with the object of depressing its functional role was DOGLIOTTI. This author, in his paper published in 1938, reports on four cases of interruption of the spinothalamic tract in order to relieve pain "at the highest level of the pons." He employed an occipitoparietal supratentorial craniotomy for this purpose. However, it is almost certain from the description presented in his paper, that destruction by means of an electrocoagulation needle was in reality performed in the postcollicular part of the mesencephalon, in the distal section of the lateral sulcus mesencephali. This conviction is also shared by BAILEY-GLEES-OPPENHEIMER who refer to DOGLIOTTI's operations in their paper published in 1954. However, the true pioneering work as regards open surgery in the region of the mesencephalon was done by EARL WALKER. This author, after a series of operations on monkeys and extensive neuroanatomic and histologic studies, discovered the probable topographic arrangement of the spinothalamic and quintothalamic tracts in the mesencephalon and determined, in his opinion, the most suitable place and extent of the incision required to produce hemianalgesia of the entire contralateral half of the body in man. He believed that the optimal site, which may be approached by the occipital supra-transtentorial route, is the intercollicular region. These interventions had an excellent effect on preoperative pain and also WALKER's approach though still very exacting appeared, in the writer's opinion based on experiences gained with 14 patients, the best and least damaging used so far. However, many further authors who, after the publication of WALKER's paper in 1942, tried his method, saw many complications which in a high percentage had to be blamed on the way of approach to the mesencephalon. Moreover, a majority of neurosurgeons testing mesencephalic tractotomy for intractable pain stated a much higher percentage incidence of postoperative hyperpathias than mentioned by WALKER.

Soon after I was put in charge of the neurosurgical section by the director of the surgical department, Prof. V. RAPANT in 1949, I came to realise that neurosurgery comprises some attractive chapters, satisfying and efficacious, as well as some unrewarding, difficult ones offering little hope. To the second category belonged at that time in our center the radical treatment of intractable pain, mainly that originating in the upper part of the body.

My endeavour was to introduce in this field full of problems all new, justifiable and recognized methods, according to the tradition of Prof. RAPANT's department. I made a thorough study of the contemporary literature on operations on the brain stem as recently advocated: I tried out medullary tractotomy, however, the overall result was not very satisfactory. In another two patients I attempted the performance of WALKER's mesencephalic tractotomy. I failed in the first female patient on account of major venous hemorrhage, occurring already during the approach to the tentorial incisura. This hemorrhage originated from a torn vein ascending to the tentorium, resulting in oedema of the exposed brain tissue. In the second case, likewise a female, I encountered an extensive venous plexus in the region of the tentorial notch and quadrigeminal bodies. After these operations in 1953 and 1954 I became convinced that these failures were due not only to my modest experience and imperfections of surgical technique, but also to the great structural obstacles encountered. These were surmounted, frequently at considerable risk, only when using the surgical approach to the quadrigeminal bodies. This was, in any case, revealed by the papers of various writers (BAILEY, WHITE and SWEET). In another two patients, for the reasons just given, I made a decision to use bilateral frontal lobotomy. Both patients were receiving high doses of opiates on account of severe pain in the upper part of the body. However, the operation resulted in the emergence of severe mental disturbances with a grave and permanent change of personality.

These bitter experiences convinced me of the fact that we did not possess a surgical method capable of suppressing pain in the upper part of the body, at the same time sufficiently satisfactory for the critical surgeon and conferring adequate relief to the patient. It is not surprising, therefore, that the admission of patients suffering from severe pains located in the upper extremities and neck was highly unwelcome to us at that time. It revealed our helplessness in this field and we had to admit to the public that so far no suitable method offering hope of radical success was available for controlling such pain.

I felt sure that these patients could not as yet be dealt with by the average skilled neurosurgeon. Such cases, if operation was carried out, were more an object of experimental interest of the neurosurgeon, than offered a real chance of improving their lot. The only operation acceptable to a degree in this hopeless situation was WALKER's mesencephalic tractotomy. His statistical results showing that only one out of fourteen operation cases died and that dysaesthesia emerged in only 10%, appeared trustworthy, despite the fact that other workers did not achieve equally excellent results with the operation. The stereotactic operations were in the initial stage at that time and experiences with them in the treatment of intractable pain were only fragmentary (SPIEGEL and WYCIS, TALAIRACH et al.).

In order to reduce the incidence of complications due to the occipital way of approach recommended by WALKER, GUIOT and FORJAZ (1947) shifted the site further to the front, the subtemporal supratentorial region. Their main object was to avoid interference with and ligation of the venous system of Labbé.

The present author during the 1954—1956 period devised a personal technique of infratentorial approach to the region of the posterior incisura. This was an accidental result of an operation in a girl aged eight years done in September 1954. The clinical pattern of the condition and pneumoventriculography had aroused suspicion of the presence of an expanding lesion in the posterior cranial fossa. Surgical exploration of the fourth ventricle, vermis and both hemispheres produced a negative result. However, both cerebellar hemispheres were pushed backwards and downwards and this offered an opportunity also for a technically simple exploration in the region of the upper surface of the cerebellar hemispheres and vermis. Both hemispheres became depressed still further and the whole region of the posterior cisterna ambiens was exposed after dissection of arachnoid folds and several bridging veins. An inoperable astroblastoma filled the whole region.

At that time I was ignorant of the paper published in 1913 by KRAUSE who devised an approach to the pineal region through the infratentorial medial route from an occipitosuboccipital craniectomy, and the surgical situation described above provided the sole incentive for experimental approaches to the region done on the post-mortem table. Thus I proceeded to elaborate the details of this surgical approach by repeated experimental operations. After these preliminaries, I decided to perform mesencephalic tractotomy in a patient using the infratentorial paramedian suboccipital approach. This was a female aged 55 years with secondary deposits of cancer of the breast. The operation was done without complications and with success in April 1955. The technique of approach was further perfected and simplified afterwards, and the incision for destruction of the spinothalamic pathway was carried higher towards the borderline between mesencephalon and thalamus and into the thalamus itself. Indications for this operation were likewise extended to include tumours in the region of the corpora quadrigemina, inflammatory and other obstructions in the posterior part of the third ventricle and to operations in the substantia nigra and lateral subthalamic area in extrapyramidal disorders.

The present author's personal method of surgical approach, however, differs in principle from the technique described by KRAUSE in 1913. Operation is done from a relatively small suboccipital hemicraniectomy, whereas KRAUSE made a wide occipitosuboccipital cranial opening. The approach to the corpora quadrigemina is paramedian, the insertions of the vermis and vascular folds in the midline are not disturbed, the cerebellar hemisphere sinks spontaneously after dissection of arachnoid trabecules and ligation of one or more bridging veins.

The sinking of the cerebellar hemisphere is entirely adequate for the exploration of the region of the posterior cisterna ambiens. KRAUSE made an occipital craniotomy in order to lift the tentorium with the aid of the brain spoon. I consider this manœuvre the most damaging part of his technique, because it exerts pressure on the vascular drainage, the confluence of sinuses, thus raising considerably force and pressure. The operations of KRAUSE, one of the pioneers of neurosurgery, must be highly appreciated in any case, in view of the limited technical scope as regards simple coagulation, suction, haemostasis, antibiotics etc.

Stereotactic surgery facilitated a marked advance in destructive interventions on the basal nuclei and thalamus. It was introduced by SPIEGEL and WYCIS who in 1947 described the first stereotactic apparatus used for such operations in man. Their first interventions were directed towards destruction of the dorsomedial thalamic nucleus in psychoses. SPIEGEL and WYCIS exploited for the construction of their apparatus the facts and experiences gleaned by HORSLEY and CLARK who already in 1906 started to use a stereotactic apparatus for experimental studies of cerebellar pathways in cats. Stereotaxis as a therapeutic method for intractable pain was also first used by SPIEGEL and WYCIS in 1948. These workers performed coagulation of the spinothalamic and bulbothalamic tracts in the midbrain at the level of the superior colliculi. Soon afterwards also others commenced using stereotaxis in the treatment of pain (DAVID, TALAIRACH et al.). Apart from the intervention in the mesencephalon just mentioned, stereotactic destruction of the dorsomedial thalamic nucleus was used for suppressing pain, for the first time likewise by SPIEGEL and WYCIS. Their object was to modify the psychic reaction of the patient against the pain present. TALAIRACH et a., since the year 1948, have been performing destruction of the end-station of the spinothalamic tract in the thalamus, the nucleus ventrocaudalis together with centrum medianum nucleus. This operation was done mainly in persons suffering from thalamic pain. Numerous other workers followed suit in destruction of the ventrocaudal nucleus and its neighbourhood, by means of stereotactic apparatus. The Freiburg school headed by RIECHERT elaborated this technique most systematically.

This last mentioned surgical technique drew our attention, when we realized from experiences gained by the preceding operations in the region of the tentorial notch that the infratentorial technique of approach facilitates easy access to the posterior thalamic and subthalamic structures. Visualization of the most distal parts of the thalamus, the medial geniculate body, is sufficient, the same applies to the tectothalamic junction. Experimental work on the midbrain and thalamus revealed that the optimal site for introduction of the needle for destruction lies at a point where both brachia colliculorum and the medial geniculate body meet. The special scalpel with a sliding loop is introduced at this juncture which is easily visualized at operation. The nuclei ventrocaudalis parvocellularis lateralis and medialis, as well as some nuclei of the truncothalamic system, with zona incerta of subthalamus are located immediately in front of the point in question. Recently we have been performing also partial destruction of the frontothalamic pathways by a personal method of the present writer designated "partial longitudinal thalamotomy."

E. WALKER in 1949 recommended still another open operation in the mesencephalon, i.e. in its cerebral peduncle. This is the so-called pedunculotomy which he performed in some types of hyperkinesia. The rationale for this was, that pathological tremor can be influenced solely by operations on the pyramidal tract, and that in this mesencephalic region the destruction of the corticospinal fibers does not produce a permanent motor deficit. Although some neurosurgeons have good experiences with this destruction of the corticospinal tract in the cerebral peduncle (WALKER, BUCY) this operation, using a temporal intradural approach, was never widely applied, because further experimental and clinical research revealed that tremor may be modified also without any involvement of voluntary motor activity by interventions in some areas of basal grey structures.

Operations for extrapyramidal disorders are at present done almost exclusively by stereotactic means. The sites that have so far proved most advantageous for these interventions are the globus pallidus, or another thalamic section, i.e. its ventrooral anterior and posterior nucleus. Destruction of this nucleus was proposed in the year 1951 by the Freiburg school and achieved wide application in later years (COOPER et al.). However, in 1958 and 1959 the well-known pioneer of open operations for extrapyramidal diseases, R. MEYERS, in collaboration with FRY and co-workers first introduced the so-called ultrasonic procedures on human brain, destroying in some cases by sound also the substantia nigra in the mesencephalon and its immediate neighbourhood. He discovered that this procedure had an equally excellent effect on the rigidity of parkinsonism, as the previously mentioned operations and that tremor is suppressed even more perfectly. These facts made me decide, in 1960, to perform nigrotomy, or lateral subthalamotomy by the open infratentorial route, thus avoiding amongst others the need for purchasing the expensive ultrasonic apparatus. A similar operation, but using an occipital transtentorial approach, was tested by RAND. Results achieved by these operations offer great hopes. Recently the advantages of the aforementioned subthalamotomy in extrapyramidal diseases, i. e. destruction of the zona incerta and Forel's field H, have been increasingly emphasized. These structures likewise may be approached by the infratentorial route. They are situated laterally from those structures which we interrupt in pain, they are, however, at only a few millimetres distance from the trigonum surface, visible during the operation.

Intractable pain and extrapyramidal disorders form thus the bulk of diseases for which at present operations on mesencephalon and thalamus are indicated. Whereas access to the mesencephalon is either by open operation or stereotactically, the various thalamic areas, apart from the personal infratentorial approach mentioned, can be reached only stereotactically. Both the available methods of access to these structures have been elaborated in detail to the present date. The risk of using them and surgical mortality are minimal. Both of them, however, offer certain advantages and have some shortcomings, increased danger and contraindications. It depends on the condition of the patient and no less on the experience of the neurosurgeon which of the two methods, stereotactic or open, is selected for treatment of pain. This question will be dealt with in the following chapters.

The history of operations on mesencephalon and thalamus, though relatively short, is already rich in its details and highly varied. Operations on structures located at great depth and very unfavourably, were devised not only on account of the neurosurgeon's mission to assist those who suffer from disease originated in this situation or capable of being modified by intervention there, but also from the wish to contribute in ever increasing measure to the knowledge of the physiological mysteries of the central nervous system. This combination of experimental and therapeutic mission of the neurosurgeon is of particularly great significance in this field at present.

III. The Anatomy and Physiology of the Mesencephalon and Thalamus from the Viewpoint of Surgical Control of Pain

Our incomplete knowledge of the anatomical-physiological facts concerning pain undoubtedly provides a stumbling block for its neurosurgical control. So far we have not been able to elucidate whether this most complicated and complex sensation is performed primarily in the receptor elements, pain fibres of the periphery, spinal cord, brain stem, or in the thalamosubcortical and cortical structures. So far we have found out in blurred outline that the sensation of pain arises from irritation of certain nervous systems, whose involvement alters sometimes disadvantageously, sometimes however favourably, the experience of pain. These systems, getting more complicated on their way towards their subcortical and cortical termination, are interrupted at present for therapeutic reasons at different sites. The region of mesencephalon and thalamus offers many obstacles from this angle. Advances in the field of therapeutic interventions are for this reason very slow in this region, determined and guided by perfection in technique, as well as by continuing discoveries in the field of neurophysiology, histology and other disciplines.

The neurosurgeon, however, in his radical fight against pain does not limit himself to the role of therapist. Each therapeutic intervention on the pain system has to-day its highly significant scientific and research component. It is desirable for these reasons that anybody who decides to perform such operations for the relief of pain in the region of the brain stem, should be well acquainted with contemporary knowledge on structure and function.

1. The Anatomy and Physiology of the Midbrain

The mid-brain, mesencephalon, is in man the smallest part of the brain, measuring only 15 to 20 mm. in length, composed of five parts altogether: telencephalon, diencephalon, mesencephalon, metencephalon and myelencephalon (Fig. 1).

The dorsal part of the mesencephalon consisting mainly of the plate of the corpora quadrigemina and possessing an architecture similar to that of the cerebral cortex, is called tectum. Its ventral part consists of the cerebral peduncles, also called crura cerebri. This ventral part is divided into the tegmentum—the internal, dorsal portion of the peduncles—and the most ventral portion, called pes pedunculi.

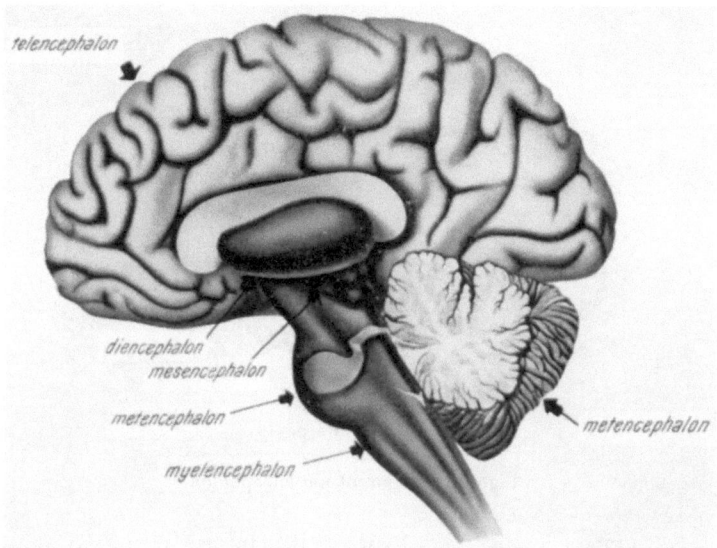

Fig. 1. Division of brain into five parts

A narrow channel connecting the third and fourth cerebral ventricles runs through the middle of the tegmentum, this is called the aqueduct of Sylvius or iter. The cerebral peduncles emerge as massive bundles of fibres from the rostral part of the pons and create between themselves in the mid-line a space called fossa interpeduncularis, or also intercruralis. Many fine perforations are situated in its roof, substantia perforata posterior, containing some of the vessels supplying the mesencephalon (Fig. 2).

The lateral groove, sulcus mesencephali lateralis, has acquired importance from the neurosurgical angle. It may be visualized from the dorsal aspect and separates the tegmentum from the peduncles on the surface. The superficial portion of the tegmentum extending from the lateral sulcus mesencephali to the inferior colliculi and their brachia consists of fibres of the so-called lateral lemniscus and is called trigonum lemnisci. This is the point of attack in WALKER's mesencephalic tractotomy for pain. Both colliculi, the superior and inferior, are still, even in man, functionally linked with thalamic nuclei by pathways creating an oblique prominence on the surface, called brachium colliculi. The brachium of the inferior colliculus runs towards the most distal thalamic nucleus, the medial geniculate body, which represents the last functional relay station of the acoustic pathway to the highest centers. Its transection during WALKER's

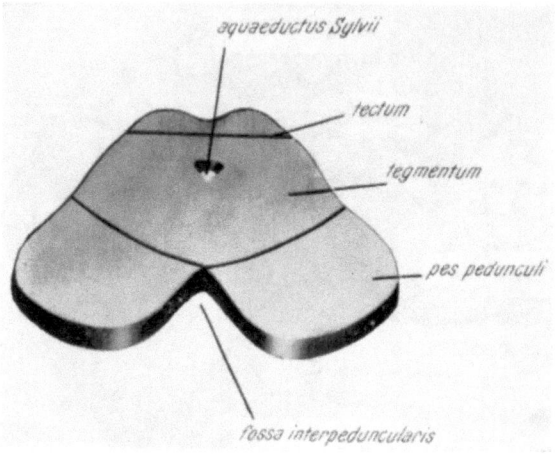

Fig. 2. Partition of mesencephalon

mesencephalic tractotomy results, accordingly, in impairment of hearing. The brachium of the superior colliculus directs its fibres to another thalamic nucleus, lateral geniculate body, situated distal and more lateral to it and conducting the secondary optic tract. The relatively small function of serving as an optical reflex centre is awarded to the superior colliculus in man. Its primary function being reflex adjustment of eyes and head to optical stimuli. In lower vertebrates, fishes and amphibia, however, it represents the main suprasegmental correlation centre (Fig. 3).

We are able to distinguish, on a cross section of the mesencephalon at the level of the inferior colliculi, the mass of the tegmentum whose uppermost part contains the crossing fibres of the so-called brachium conjunctivum from the superior cerebellar peduncle; further, we find there pyramidal and corticopontine fibres, constituents of the pes pedunculi and dorsally from these a darkish brown elongated band of nuclear structure called substantia nigra. Fibres of the lateral lemniscus surround and enter the inferior colliculus, representing functionally the secondary pathway for hearing.

The medial and paramedial structures of the mesencephalon, the region surrounding the aqueduct and situated ventrally from it, are

composed of a large number of grey nuclei and long, interposed
tracts also crossing there: the functional role of these structures is
important, albeit complex and much of it remains to be elucidated.
The neurosurgeon is aware of the colossal importance of this region

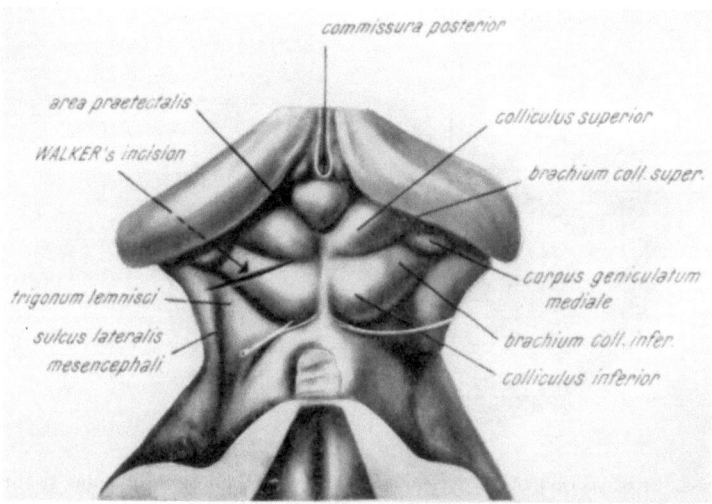

Fig. 3. Superficial structures of dorsum of mesencephalon. From F. KOPSCH: Lehrbuch und Atlas der Anatomie des Menschen, Bd. III. Leipzig: G. Thieme. 1953

in connection with operative probing of the aqueduct. He knows
that creation of a "fausse route" during this delicate procedure
results in a severe postoperative course and frequently also in the
death of the patient from progressive oedema of these paramedial
centres and the reticular formation of the mesencephalon.

The paramedial region of the mesencephalon has not so far been
the centre of direct neurosurgical interest for the reasons just
suggested. It seems hardly feasible to make therapeutic interventions here by using the crude technique generally employed at present for destruction of other areas of the midbrain or grey nuclei,
regardless of whether we entertain the thought of stereotaxis or
open operation. Perhaps at a time when the technique of stimulation or destruction of a small number of cells will be available,
interest in the question of therapeutic interventions in this region
will be revived, particularly if we are convinced that an important
part of fibres conducting painful stimuli terminate there. For this
reason also "medial" mesencephalotomy proposed recently by
ROEDER and ORTHNER must be done to a very limited extent and

on one side only, if it is not to result in impairment of consciousness and other vital signs.

The so-called central grey matter surrounds the aqueduct, its caudal and ventral portion contains the nucleus of the fourth

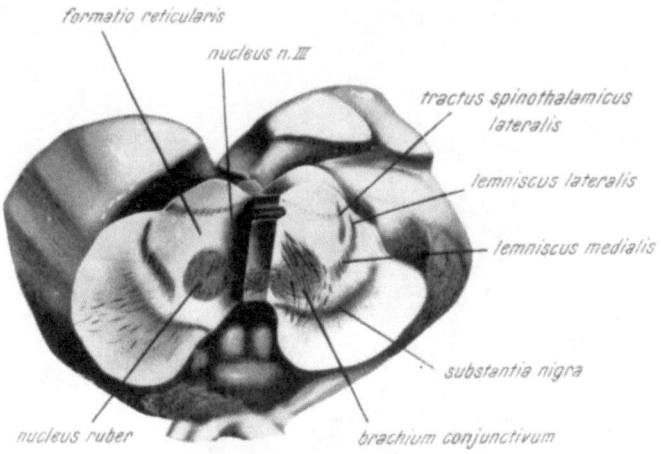

Fig. 4. Cross-section of mesencephalon at level of inferior colliculus (right) and superior colliculus (left)

cranial nerve. The medial longitudinal fasciculus runs ventrally from this nucleus, containing ascending and descending fibres. It is a relay station particularly for part of the ocular innervation, nervus abducens and nervus oculomotorius. Even more ventrally is the already mentioned decussation of the brachium conjunctivum (Fig. 4, on right).

The cross-section made at the level of the superior colliculi (Fig. 4, on left), shows a new structure, the nucleus ruber, as a continuation of one already crossed portion of the brachium conjunctivum and further the nuclear complex of the III. cranial nerve. Nucleus ruber here occupies a large part of the tegmentum. It has afferent and efferent paths, forming a functional link between cerebellum and premotor and motor cortex. It is an important centre where extrapyramidal impulses from cortex, thalamus and striatum are relayed to the motor neurons of stem and spinal cord. The nuclear complex of the III. cranial nerve has an elongated shape in a craniocaudal direction, it is situated in the ventral part of the central grey matter. It is composed of three main nuclei, n. centralis, n. Edinger-Westphal and n. medialis anterior. Finally, here also commences the so-called central tegmental tract, situated in the reticular formation of the tegmentum and containing descending fibres, terminating mainly in the olive. This is well developed in man. Its functional role has not yet been fully elucidated, possibly it represents a link in an evolutionally more recent path connecting corpus striatum and thalamus with the cerebellum.

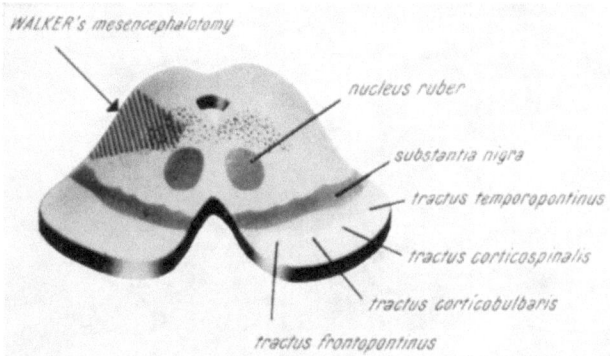

Fig. 5. Cross-section of mesencephalon with WALKER's incision

Still further in a cephalad direction from the third nerve nuclei at the level of the juncture between third ventricle and aqueduct lies the interstitial nucleus of Cajal, immediately dorsally from it the Darkschewitsch nucleus. Both belong functionally to the extrapyramidal system too.

The junction between mesencephalon and thalamus is created dorsally by the so-called pretectal area. This is a centre for pupillary reflexes (RANSON and MAGOUN). In the region of this pretectal area, at the junction of the third ventricle and aqueduct, a small bundle of crossing and obliquely coursing fibres forms the dorsal wall creating the so-called posterior commissure. Its fibres connect numerous cellular structures of the basal and stem ganglia. Some spinothalamic fibres also penetrate it running towards the opposite thalamus and subthalamus.

The substantia nigra is the largest nuclear mass of the mesencephalon. It runs throughout its whole length towards the diencephalon. Of all mammals it is most developed in man. It is an important centre of the extrapyramidal system, possibly a relay system between pyramidal and extrapyramidal paths. For this reason it has caught, in recent years, the interest of a so far narrow circle of neurosurgeons. Thanks to MEYERS, FRY and others, its destruction achieves good results in some extrapyramidal disorders. Substantia nigra thus takes its place besides the globus pallidus,

pallidofugal paths and thalamic nucleus ventrooralis, or lateral subthalamic area, as a site where the neurosurgeon is able to influence
the manifestations of extrapyramidal diseases.

Corticospinal and corticobulbar paths run in the central three
fifths of the pes pedunculi, frontopontine paths in the medial portion

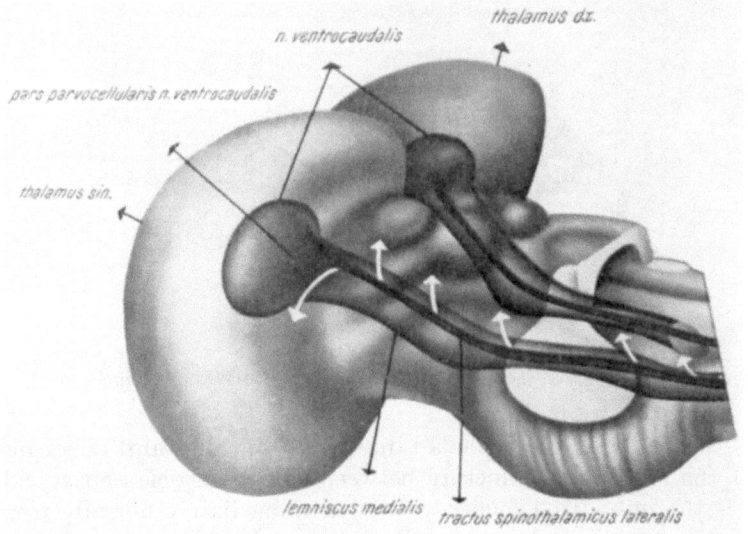

Fig. 6. Drawing showing course of medial lemniscus and spinothalamic tract through
medulla and stem

of this structure, in its lateral part temporoparietooccipitopontine
paths. The existing results have shown that the corticospinal fibres
in the cerebral peduncles are segregated from all ascending and
descending multineuronal pathways, contrary to the region of the
internal capsule, spinal cord etc. For this reason their destruction
in the pes pedunculi does not result in a complex picture of permanent motor deficit. BUCY and others exploit these experiences
for sections of the central portion of the peduncle in some extrapyramidal disorders (Fig. 5).

The medial lemniscus (Fig. 6) is an important afferent structure
traversing the mesencephalon. This is a broad bundle of fibres
composed of various sensory elements. The bundle at its entry into
the mesencephalon lies parallel with the substantia nigra, dorsally
from it. In its further cranial course it is deflected so that its lateral
margin is directed dorsally, forming an angular knee-like bend resulting in the shift of its medial section as far ventrally as possible

(Fig. 4). Its fibres are a continuation of the Goll and Burdach bundles ascending from the periphery and projecting impulses from proprioceptive and specific tactile end organs to the ventrocaudal thalamic nucleus. It also contains the ventral spinothalamic tract, whose path of tactile sensation has not yet been fully understood.

2. The Course of the Pain Tract in the Medulla and Brain Stem

The lateral spinothalamic tract as a "specific" secondary afferent pathway for pain and temperature (Fig. 6), commences in the posterior horns of the cord and partially crosses in the anterior spinal commissure. It lies in the lower section of the mesencephalon with its main bundle slightly dorsally and dorso-laterally from the lateral margin of the medial lemniscus. However, here, according to Kuru, it is mixed with fibres from the lateral lemniscus. The spinothalamic bundle, from the border of both colliculi, adjoins the dorsal margin of the medial lemniscus, underneath the brachium of the inferior colliculus. Thus it runs up to the level of the medial geniculate body, lying immediately medially and ventrally from it. At the mesencephalothalamic junction into the so-called porta thalami after Hassler, the fibres of the spinothalamic bundle divide into a medial and lateral bundle (Bowsher, 1961). Afterwards these terminate in various posterior and basal parts of the thalamic nuclei. The so-called spinotectal tract conducting also afferent pain and temperature stimuli is deflected from the spinothalamic bundle whilst traversing the mesencephalon. After previously forming a common tract, it now rotates dorso-medially and terminates at the superior and inferior colliculus. For this reason the tract is also designated as spinocollicular.

Painful sensation from the region of the face and its organs is transmitted mainly by the fifth cranial nerve and also by some fibres of n, VII, IX and X (Fig. 7, after Kunc and Maršala, 1962). It is conducted by the secondary bulbothalamic tract, thus corresponding to the spinothalamic tract for the remaining parts of the body. It originates from the nucleus of the descending trigeminal path at the medullospinal junction, known in connection with Sjöqvist's tractotomy. The term "bulbothalamic" tract is more fitting than "quintothalamic", or "trigeminothalamic", in view of the already mentioned fact that this tract contains pain fibres also from nerves other than the fifth cranial nerve.

The ascending course of this tract was determined by Wallenberg already in the year 1896 and his findings are valid with some minor alterations up to the present day. This author found that the fibres of the bulbothalamic tract divide at the pontomesencephalic border, located on this level near the dorso-lateral margin of the reticular formation. During their further course in the mesencephalon they continue to lie very paramedially, not far from the central periaqueductal grey substance, i.e. very deeply. The mesencephalic

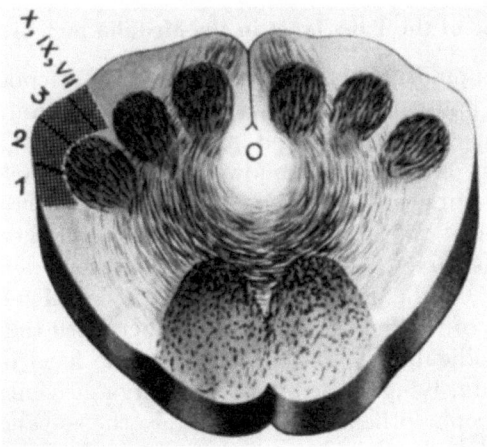

Fig. 7. Localization of pain fibres belonging to spinal trigeminal tract, n. VII, IX and X in the lower medulla

section of the bulbothalamic tract lies medially and somewhat ventrally from the lateral spinothalamic bundle, its destruction at this level requires an incision at least 5 mm. in depth. Ipsilateral, i.e. uncrossed bulbothalamic fibres in relatively great numbers are found, according to LANDGREN, in the region of the central tegmental tract.

These findings of WALLENBERG detected in rats and later verified in man by CRAWFORD, GLEES and others as well as by our personal experience with mesencephalic tractotomy, appear to be correct and disagree with WALKER's findings in monkeys. WALKER found degeneration of bulbothalamic fibres only 2 mm. beneath the surface, immediately dorsally from the lateral mesencephalic sulcus. Such an incision does not result in the slightest impairment of sensibility in the face.

The "direct" fibres conducting pain and temperature are arranged segmentally already in the spinal cord (PETREN, 1910). Dorsally and laterally situated fibres are for the lower body segments, whereas fibres belonging to the upper body segments are located ventrally and more medially. This somatotopic arrangement is maintained in the mesencephalon (WALKER, 1940) and the thalamus (LE GROS CLARK, 1937). However, a small number of these fibres is mixed up haphazardly (WALKER). The arrangement of bulbothalamic fibres, situated as mentioned already, medially from the spinothalamic tract, is similar: mandibular, maxillary and ophthalmic branches are arranged in dorsoventral sequence (STOPFORD, 1925; McKINLEY and MAGOUN, 1942, etc.). They are also joined by pain fibres of the VII., IX. and X. cranial nerves.

Neurosurgical practice does not exploit—on a larger scale—this topographic arrangement of specific pain fibres for their destruction. This is difficult in the region of the midbrain in view of the limited extent of the spinothalamic tract, even though some writers report such isolated destruction of only part of the spinothalamic bundle in the mesencephalon (GUIOT and FORJAZ, 1947; BAILEY-GLEES and OPPENHEIMER, 1954). Also some of the present writer's operations had as their object the interruption of the pain pathway of only certain body segments. Of course, for lasting relief, such procedures cannot be realized accurately, because of the great diffusion of direct and indirect pain fibres in the brain stem. Also at thalamic nuclear termination the individual body regions have their representation of sensibility spread over a larger area of posterior thalamic nuclei.

The face forms a surgical exception in that respect. Using a specific technique, FALCONER, later KUNC in our country and others, perform only partial selective tractotomies of the spinal (primary) trigeminal tract below the level of obex, with great and permanent success (Fig. 7).

The described "specific" spinothalamic tract does not, of course, represent by far the total afferent system of pain. GLEES and BAILEY found at the level of the superior colliculi only about 1500 pain fibres, two thirds of which had a diameter of 2—4 microns, the remainder as a rule 4—6 microns. The fibres were at this level concentrated in a small compact cord occupying an area of only approximately 0.65 mm². Although experiences with mesencephalic tractotomy show that also these direct long fibres are arranged on a wider section than was ascertained by GLEES and BAILEY, nevertheless these findings reveal that a reduction of a great number of fibres in the spinothalamic bundle takes place during its ascending course through the brain stem. Numerous fibres detach themselves from this bundle in the medulla, pons and midbrain and course towards the more medial structures of the stem. CHANG and RUCH, MORUZZI and MAGOUN, BRODAL, WALBERG and BLACKSTAD, MORIN, SCHWARTZ and O'LEARY, GARDNER and MORIN, MEHLER, BOW-

SHER and others are amongst the prominent writers who showed by their electrophysiological and histological studies that there exist also other structures conducting painful and, as the case may be, other sensoric impulses, in the medulla and midbrain, thus creating

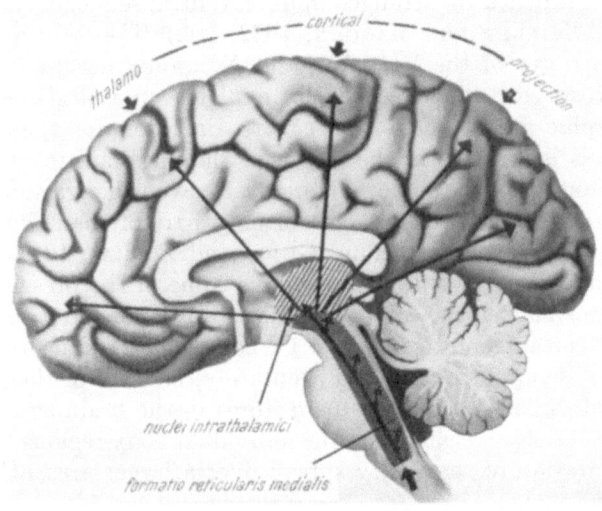

Fig. 8. Approximate extent and projection of reticular formation. Partially from F. H. NETTER: The CIBA Collection of Medical Illustrations. Vol. 1: Nervous System. Published by CIBA, 1957

some indirect paths for pain and other qualities of sensibility. Of these, the ascending reticular system (FÖRSTER and GAGEL, 1932) is by far the most important (Fig. 8).

The reticular formation represents a network of nerve fibres and nuclei occupying wide areas of the medulla, pons and mesencephalon. Though not yet possessing entirely precise histological and physiological borders, it appears certain that it extends structurally and from a functional aspect for a much wider area in a rostral as well as caudal direction. Already in the spinal cord there are numerous cells, mainly surrounding the central canal, not belonging to either the motor or sensory systems of the anterior or posterior horns of grey spinal substance. There is an ever increasing number of these cells in a cranial direction. This cellular system is continued in the medial part of the reticular formation in the medulla. Similarly, at the cranial extremity, cells of the reticular formation are identical in their structure and role with cells of the intralaminar group of thalamic nuclei.

Facts discovered so far show that the reticular system may be divided into a lateral and medial part. The lateral part is short and limited to the section of the stem only. According to a majority of writers, this lateral part does not contain any long fibres, though VALVERDE in 1961 found there also long axones, taking a rostral course. Otherwise this section is connected by short axones with the medial reticular formation. Cells of the medial formation send out axones either rostrally creating the for us important so-called ascending reticular system, or caudally, or finally they might divide into ascending and descending rami. From the ascending reticular system impulses are relayed to the intralaminar thalamic nuclei, finally reaching the cortex by diffuse thalamocortical projection (MORIN et al., 1951; BOWSHER, 1961).

Part of the ascending reticular pathway is made up also from fibres detached from the spinothalamic bundle during its course through the medulla and brain stem. It has not yet been decided whether the tract thus produced should be considered a mere collateral of the long ascending tracts, or as an independent medial spinoreticular tract. Experimental studies by SPIVY and METCALF in 1959 and MEHLER-FEFERMAN and NAUTA in 1960 incline more to the opinion that they represent, basically, entirely independent systems of fibres.

Termination of fibres of the ascending reticular system takes place either in one of the reticular nuclei of the medulla, or brain stem, or not till the intralaminar thalamic nuclei. Many of these ascending fibres were discovered in the reticular nuclei of the mesencephalon, either in the paramedial sections of the reticular formation of the tegmentum, or also in the periaqueductal grey substance and finally in the region dorsally from the nucleus ruber. As far as the spinothalamic fibres are concerned, some traverse the reticular formation of the stem and return again to the spinothalamic bundle, others terminate in the reticular nuclei of the stem, and finally others run as far as the thalamic nuclei. In the region of the mesencephalon this applies mainly to the periaqueductal grey substance with the so-called nucleus tegmenti pedunculopontinus, interstitial nucleus and nucleus paralemniscalis, which receive fibres from the spinothalamic tract (BOWSHER, 1957). MEHLER-FEFERMAN and NAUTA, however, were unable to find in the two last mentioned nuclei terminations of spinothalamic fibres. That group of fibres which runs towards the periaqueductal grey substance is, according to BAILEY and DAVIS in 1944 and HUNSPERGER in 1956 and others, responsible for the origin of affective reactions to painful stimuli.

Pain fibres, which terminate in the nuclei of the reticular formation of the mesencephalon or traverse it, may project further into
the thalamus, as a rule on the same side, or may also traverse by
the posterior commissure to the contralateral thalamus (CHANG and
RUCH, 1947, in monkeys; BOWSHER, 1957, in man). Some fibres
mainly from the sections of the stem lying closely paramedially also
enter the subthalamus, the hypothalamus, or the globus pallidus.
The descending portion of the reticular formation is not directly
connected with pain conduction, though even in this respect recent
findings by BRODAL (1957) are very interesting: a majority of long
descending axones of the reticular formation have their origin
rostrally from the origin of the zone of ascending axones (TORVIK
and BRODAL, 1957). Ascending axones thus traverse the field of
neurones projecting caudally and vice versa. BRODAL, therefore,
believes that ascending and descending reticular impulses are mu-
tually directly correlated functionally.

It may be stated in conclusion that pain conduction in the medulla and brain stem is transmitted on the one hand by the "specific" spinothalamic tract, spinotectal and also by the long spino-
reticulospinothalamic tracts, by spinoreticulothalamic fibres and
finally by monosynaptic or polysynaptic links or tracts connecting
the spinothalamic with the reticulothalamic tracts. Some of these
fibres traverse to the opposite side even in the upper stem by the
posterior commissure. This complexity of pain conduction is blamed
for the existence of various qualities of pain and for the origin of
various "pathological" pains after only a partial interruption of
afferent pain pathways. At the same time this illustrates the highly
difficult situation confronting the neurosurgeon in his endeavour
to influence the pain impulses by operation in the brain stem.

3. The Blood Supply of the Mesencephalon

It is important to be thoroughly cognizant with the blood supply
to the mesencephalon and with vascular topography particularly
as regards open operations, though the danger of damaging these
vessels is much more real in stereotactic operations and, what is
more, not capable of control.

WALKER, already in his first papers on mesencephalic tractotomy
for pain published in the years 1940 and 1942, draws attention to the
possible presence of an extensive network of voluminous veins,
making the approach to the corpora quadrigemina difficult or preventing it altogether. These drainage veins form even normally a
fine, dense network in the pia mater and open into the basal veins.

The venous blood from there enters Galen's vein, or the internal cerebral vein. If the venous network over the corpora quadrigemina is too dense, or if it consists of dilated closely accumulated veins, their dissection may be become dangerous particularly because the arterial blood supply might be interfered with at the same time.

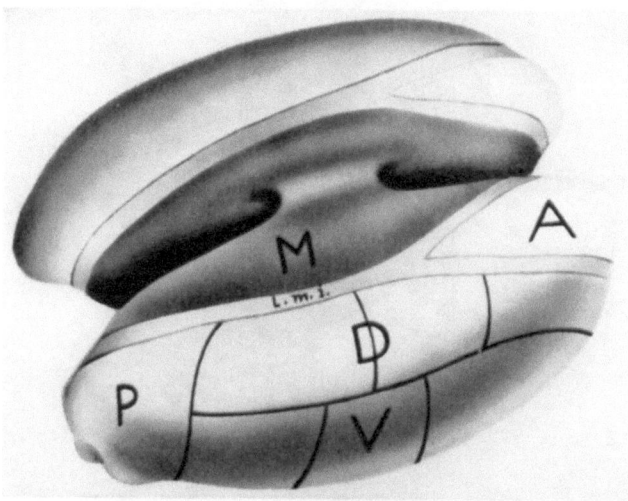

Fig. 9. Thalamus and its groups of nuclei. From F. H. NETTER: The CIBA Collection of Medical Illustrations, Vol. I: Nervous System. Published by CIBA, 1957

The region of the corpora quadrigemina receives its blood supply from the quadrigeminal arteries, branches of the posterior cerebral artery. Apart from this, small branches from the superior cerebellar artery and the posterior chorioidal artery run towards the dorsum of the mesencephalon. The lateral part of the tegmentum, substantia nigra and external part of pes pedunculi receive their blood supply by short branches from the posterior cerebral and superior cerebellar arteries. Medial and paramedial structures of the midbrain, including medial longitudinal fasciculus, and nucleus ruber, are supplied by vessels penetrating the posterior perforated substance in the interpeduncular fossa. These vessels are branches of the arteria communicans posterior and arteria cerebri posterior.

4. The Anatomy and Physiology of the Thalamus

The thalamus (Fig. 9) is the main terminal station of secondary pain pathways. A smaller percentage of fibres conducting pain impulses enter directly the subthalamus and a tiny number the hypothalamus and the globus pallidus too.

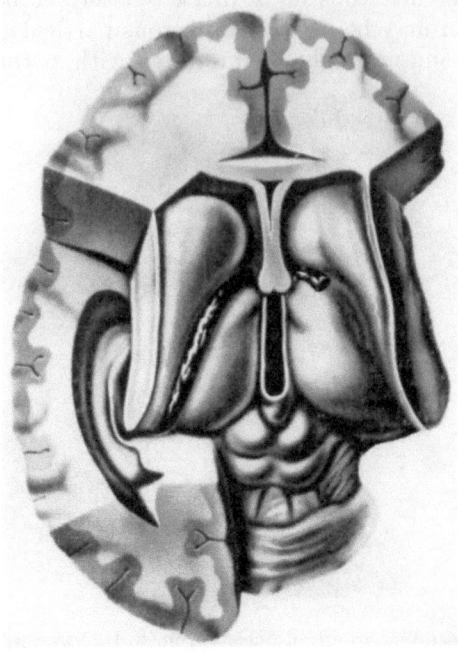

Fig. 10. Relations of both thalami to neighbourhood. From F. H. NETTER: The CIBA Collection of Medical Illustrations, Vol. I: Nervous System. Published by CIBA. 1957

The thalamus constitutes an extensive nuclear structure of irregular, ovoid shape, forming the largest i.e. dorsal portion of the diencephalon. Its ventral portion constitutes the larger hypothalamus, lying medioventrally and the smaller subthalamus, or ventral thalamus lying laterally. Both halves of the thalamus are located in front closer to the midline and are separated there only by the space created by the anterior part of the third ventricle. They are more widely separated at the rear and create a larger space between themselves containing the pineal gland and the superior colliculi of the midbrain. Length and height are of individual size in man. Differences are only small as a rule, however, they have to be taken into account with stereotactic operations. TALAIRACH reports, in connection with these operations, in his paper published in 1955, the maximal possible difference in outer length of the thalamus as 7,5 mm. with a mean length of 35.25 mm. and the maximal difference in height possible as 5 mm. with a mean of 16.5 mm. (Fig. 10).

As far as the terminology of individual sections and nuclei of the thalamus is concerned, terms according to C. and O. Vogt (1941) will be mainly used, as supplemented and altered by Hassler. With important nuclear structures, mention is made also of designations after Le Gros Clark (1932) and Walker (1938) for comparison.

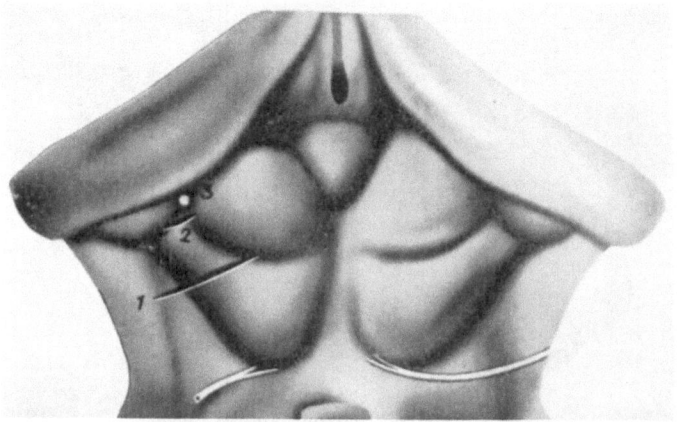

Fig. 11. Site and extent of antalgic incisions in mesencephalon and at mesence-phalothalamic juncture. *1* intercollicular Walker's mesencephalotomy, *2* "upper" mesencephalotomy, *3* the point of contact of brachia-c.g.m. Partially from F. Kopsch: Lehrbuch und Atlas der Anatomie des Menschen, Bd. III. Leipzig: G. Thieme. 1953

5. Posterior Structures of the Thalamus

The thalamic structure at its lowest end is the medial geniculate body (corpus geniculatum mediale). We shall encounter it for this reason repeatedly, in connection with interventions against pain, hereafter it will be known by its initial letters c.g.m. It is entered by the lateral lemniscus containing fibres of the third order from the ipsilateral and contralateral cochlear nucleus. The so-called geniculotemporal tract originates from the c.g.m., forming the acoustic radiation traversing the internal capsule and terminating in the temporal cortex. Some writers count to the c.g.m. also the so-called nucleus medialis, or pars magnocellularis c.g.m., others regard it as the caudal part of the posterior ventral thalamic nucleus. This is probably the part which Hassler terms nucleus ventrocaudalis portae. A tiny part of the spinothalamic tract fibres terminate also in this nucleus.

C.g.m., in conjunction with another nucleus located basally and more laterally, the so-called corpus geniculatum laterale, are called

metathalamus. Corpus geniculatum laterale contains optic tract
fibres. C. g. m. with both brachia colliculorum forms on the surface
a perceptible point of contact which is the external guiding point
in thalamotomy for pain from an infratentorial approach, devised
by the present writer (Fig. 11).

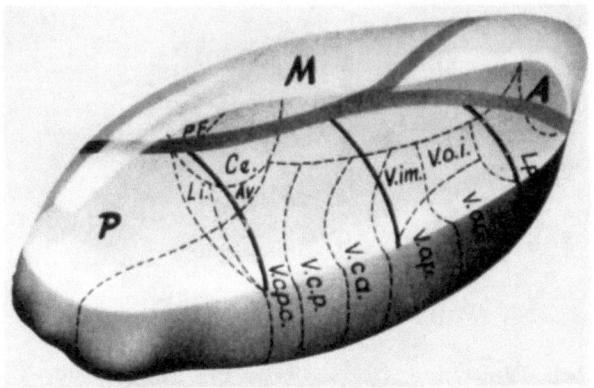

Fig. 12. Ventral thalamus and its nuclei

Another extensive part of the thalamus projects dorsally above
the metathalamus, the pulvinar. It extends still further backwards
and more laterally than the metathalamus, thus covering in rooflike
fashion the superior colliculi, pretectal area and metathalamus.
Pulvinar is one of the least investigated parts of the thalamus and
WALKER designates it in his paper on normal and pathological thalamic physiology published in 1959 as "terra ignota." We, at
present, include it with the so-called association nuclei, i. e. such
nuclei which receive exclusively intrathalamic afferent fibres and
are connected with the cortex by efferent fibres.

6. The Lateral Part of the Thalamus

The large part of the thalamus situated in front of the pulvinar
may be conveniently divided into a lateral and medial portion. Its
border is formed by a fine strand of fibres running obliquely, called
lamina medullaris interna (Figs. 9 and 12). According to POWELL
and COWAN this is the thalamic extension of the mesencephalic
reticular formation. The lateral portion, though homogenous, is
divided for reasons of functional differences into a dorsal and ventral
mass, whereas the dorsal mass continues in the pulvinar. It seems

likely that pulvinar belongs to this dorsal thalamic mass not only topographically but also as regards function.

The dorsal mass located in front of the pulvinar is called nucleus dorsalis, this gradually narrows in a frontal direction. Similarly as pulvinar, nucleus dorsalis does not appear a direct receptor nucleus, but a centre for higher integration, combination and association activities. This nucleus was subdivided by HASSLER into caudal, intermediary and oral sections. The nucleus possesses numerous internuclear links directed mainly towards ventral and medial thalamic nuclei. Nucleus dorsalis is connected with an extensive cortical section, mainly the upper parietal lobe and gyrus supramarginalis. The most forward portion of this nuclear complex is called nucleus lateropolaris by HASSLER. Despite the fact that this section also extends far dorsally, it nevertheless also comprises extrathalamic fibres and is for this reason frequently allocated to the ventral group.

The ventral group of the lateral portion of thalamic nuclei is the most important, at present, from the neurosurgical point of view. This group is also subdivided in an posterior-anterior direction into subsections, their nomenclature, however, is not uniform either. Anglo-American writers most often use the following terms: nucleus ventralis posterior (VP), n. ventralis lateralis (VL) and n. ventralis anterior (VA). HASSLER divides it into nucleus ventrocaudalis (n. v. c), n. intermedius (n. v. i.) and n. ventrooralis (n. v. o.). N. ventrocaudalis is the end station of the sensory afferent path in the thalamus. Here terminate specific tracts of medial lemniscus, lateral spinothalamic tract (Fig. 6), secondary trigeminal tract and probably also the secondary tract for taste sense. In the central part of this ventral group, i. e. the intermediary ventral nucleus, is, in all probability, the terminal station of cerebellar fibres. In the anterior part, the nucleus ventrooralis, that of fibres from the globus pallidus. The last named part of the ventral group is of paramount interest for stereotactic surgery as regards treatment of extrapyramidal disorders (RIECHERT, 1952).

7. Terminations of the Pain Tracts

The long fibres of the spinothalamic pain tract terminate, as discovered by CHANG and RUCH in 1947 only in the basal part of the aforementioned ventrocaudal nucleus. In view of the fact that this basal part of the nucleus is composed almost exclusively of small cells, in contrast to its surroundings, it is called nucleus parvocellularis by HASSLER (n. v. c. pc.). This section is called pars caudalis VP in the Anglo-American terminology. The major part of the

spinothalamic tract in man terminates at the nucleus v.c.pc., as do
also some spinoreticulothalamic fibres (BAILEY, GLEES and OPPEN-
HEIMER, 1954). HASSLER and RIECHERT (1953 and 1959) confirmed
the abovementioned localization of pain and temperature-conduct-
ing fibres in the thalamus of man by stereotactic stimulation and
destruction. Nuclear stimulation by high frequency alternating
current causes pain. The insertion of the cannula into the nucleus
also is sometimes associated with unpleasant lancinating sensations,
as observed by the present writer in several cases. MARK and ERVIN
in 1960 failed to obtain a painful response following stimulation of
VP in some of their patients, probably on account of the fact that
they failed to strike the basal part of the nucleus.

Successful attempts to strike and destroy solely the basal part
of the ventrocaudal nucleus result in the elimination or in considerable reduction of pain and temperature sensitivity, whereas tactile
and proprioceptive sensitivity remains unaffected or only slightly
impaired. This is due to the fact that medial lemniscus fibres terminate in a wide section of VP including its most dorsal and frontal
parts and that they have bilateral representation. In contrast to this
the direct fibres of the spinothalamic tract, as already referred to,
end solely in its basal part. However, termination of some long pain
fibres was also found in the most lateral part of the thalamus, the
nucleus reticularis thalami, situated close to the internal capsule.
BOWSHER (1961) allocates these fibres to the truncothalamic system
and not to the phylogenetically more recent neospinothalamic
tract.

The somatotopic arrangement of the terminations of afferent
fibres is also present in the thalamic nuclei, as repeatedly verified
experimentally and clinically (WALLENBERG, 1900; CHANG and
RUCH, 1947). This means that this segmental arrangement of spinothalamic fibres is maintained also right up to its end station in the
thalamus, however, it is spread over a more extensive area there.
These areas are already sufficiently extensive for individual parts
of the body for realistically entertaining the possibility of their
isolated destruction. Of course, the success of this limited intervention was not lasting in the majority of cases.

MOUNTCASTLE and HENNEMANN (1952) determined the exact
topographic position of individual skin segments in the ventrocaudal nucleus in monkeys by means of action potentials. HASSLER
in collaboration with RIECHERT (1959) was able to determine,
during stereotactic operations in man, centres of individual parts
of the body for pain in the nucleus, by stimulation. Here too, fibres
for the lower parts of the body are in a lateral location, whereas

representation of pain for the upper half of the body is in the medial part, also called nucleus arcuatus, or semilunaris. WALKER, however, reserves this term only for the most medial portion of nucleus ventralis posteromedialis or n. v. p. internus, probably the site where taste sense fibres terminate. Fibres of the bulbothalamic tract terminate laterally close to this part. It is also noted with interest that the mucous membrane of mouth and tongue has its final pain representation in the thalamus predominantly on the ipsilateral side, i. e. not crossed over.

Pain fibres separating from the specific spinothalamic tract on its course through the brain stem also terminate at various other sites in the thalamus, not only the n. v. c. pc. However, before dealing with their terminations, so highly important from the angle of surgical therapy, we must conclude in brief the morphological and physiological division of the thalamus.

8. The Medial Part of the Thalamus

Nucleus medialis dorsalis or territorium mediale occupies the medial part of the thalamus. This large nucleus has extensive links with a majority of the other thalamic nuclei and the periventricular grey substance. It also represents a large projection region for the prefrontal cortex. The anterior and medial parts of this nucleus project chiefly towards the gyrus rectus, area 11, the anterior lateral portion to area 47, medial central portion to area 10, lateral central portion to area 45 and 46. The posterior caudal parts of the nucleus project by medial fibres to area 9, lateral ones mainly to areas 44 and 45 (Fig. 13).

Histological investigations made in psychiatric cases submitted to frontal lobotomy by FREEMAN and WATTS revealed massive degeneration of the dorsomedial thalamic nucleus. These findings led SPIEGEL and WYCIS already in 1948 to perform destruction of the dorsomedial nucleus for intractable pain. This operation reduced emotional reactions of the patient towards pain. However, this desirable effect was accompanied by undesirable alterations of the patient's intellect. Further experiences with destruction of the dorsomedial nucleus revealed that mental defects as serious as those following bilateral frontal lobotomy frequently occur after unilateral operation (RIECHERT, ZAPLETAL). The present writer exploited the advantages of the infratentorial way of approach for performing destruction of a minor part of frontothalamic pathways in the thalamus in some instances of central pain, or in the presence of an increased emotional component. This operation on the one hand transects a part of the centrum medianum as well as eliminating those fibres of the medial nucleus which project to areas 9, 44 and possibly also 45 Brodmann's zone.

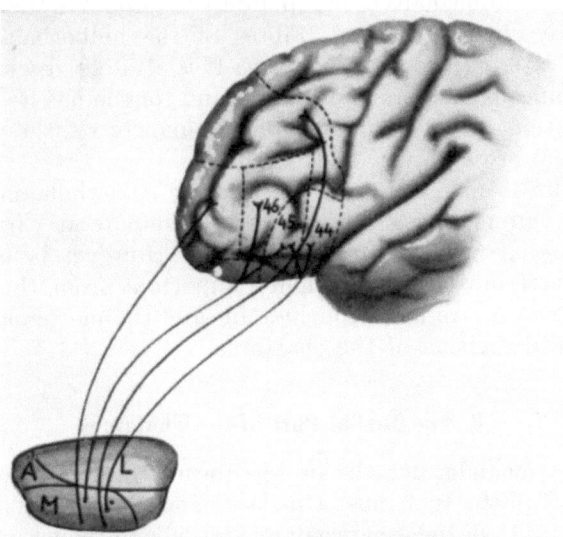

Fig. 13. Cortical projection of part of medial thalamic nucleus. From G. SCHALTEN-BRAND and P. BAILEY: Introduction to Stereotaxis with an Atlas of the Human Brain. Stuttgart: G. Thieme. 1959

9. The Truncothalamic System

A group of predominantly small ganglionic structures forms an irregular sheath throughout the lateral border of the dorsal medial nucleus extending from the rostral thalamic pole right up to the posterior commissure. It thus forms an independent structure, called involucrum mediale, whose surface border is created by the lamina medullaris interna. This involucrum mediale (HASSLER) is, according to Anglo-American writers, the most important group of the so-called truncothalamic system, comprising all those thalamic nuclei which fail to degenerate in experiments following removal of the cortex and are thus not directly dependent on the cortex (WALKER, C. and O. VOGT). The central grey substance of the thalamus under the third ventricle ependyma and ganglion habenulae, the later already part of the epithalamus, belong to the truncothalamic system, apart from the involucrum mediale.

Some fibres conducting pain also terminate in some of the nuclei comprising the involucrum mediale. These are in particular nucleus limitans at the junction of mesencephalon and thalamus, centrum medianum or central thalamic nucleus and finally its part, nucleus parafascicularis. All fibres terminating here create the main part of "subsidiary" pain pathway responsible by a majority of writers for the fact that simple destruction of n. v. c. pc. is not followed by complete relief of pain and for the origin of relapses. LE GROS CLARK in the year 1936 was the first to discover afference of myelinated fibres to the nucleus parafascicularis. According to HASSLER, some spinothalamic fibres after traversing the porta thalami end in the nucleus limitans. The existence of pain fibres in this site was confirmed also by WHITLOCK and PERL in 1959. HASSLER also found that the nucleus limitans projects with the greatest probability to the globus pallidus and is, therefore an apparent component of the primitive pain pathway, lacking cortical regulation. However, KNIGHTON already in 1950 asserted that this path also is linked with the cortical system by means of projection to the second sensitive region. Functional links between nucleus limitans and globus pallidus, however, were demonstrated also by findings at pallidotomy performed on account of extrapyramidal disorders. Stimulation of the globus pallidus was followed by registration of painful reactions. Centrum medianum is the largest nucleus of the truncothalamic system (WALKER). According to some, part of the pain fibres end here also (BOWSHER, 1957), mainly part of the bulbothalamic tract fibres. Others (LE GROS CLARK, 1937; MOUNTCASTLE, 1952; GLEES, 1953), however, believe that fibres merely traverse this nucleus and that they terminate in the adjoining nucleus arcuatus. On the whole contemporary opinion favours the centrum medianum as the main integration centre for the activities of the remaining thalamic nuclei thus assuming it to be also an important component of the subsidiary pain afference. The centrum medianum possesses very numerous short links with the reticular formation of the mesencephalon (HASSLER, KRUGER). In view of the fact that stimulation of this nucleus causes the sensation of painful fear and excitement, as found by HASSLER in man, it seems highly probable that fibres from the region of the periaqueductal grey matter terminate in this nucleus. Their function was already referred to in the morphologico-physiological chapter on the mesencephalon.

10. The Extrathalamic Terminations of Pain Fibres

Apart from the just described subsidiary pathways of pain conduction terminating in parts of the thalamus other than the VP (n. v. c. pc.), some other pain fibres by-pass the thalamus altogether. These are mainly fibres of the ventromedial portion of the reticular

formation of the midbrain, also periaqueductal grey matter fibres
with their termination in the subthalamus or hypothalamus (KAR-
PLUS and KREIDL, 1910; SPIEGEL et al., 1954; RAND et al., 1958).
Globus pallidus receives, apart from afferent fibres from the nucleus
limitans, also direct fibres from the spinothalamic tract, as discovered already by BECHTĚREV (cited HASSLER, 1960). Also the zona
incerta, which is the nuclear component of the subthalamus and,
as has already been stated, also its laterodorsal continuation, i.e.
nucleus reticularis thalami, receives part of the painful afferent
fibres. Some fibres continue from them on their course to the hypothalamus, others end here. Functionally, this group of mainly
laterally located nuclei and tracts of the subthalamus belongs to the
pallidostriatal system. The zona incerta lying medially and ventrally
is together with the Forel area H_1 injured in open thalamotomy.
It was revealed that destruction of these structures to the extent
described, is not followed by any perceptible extrapyramidal functional disturbances.

The terminations of pain conduction in other structures of diencephalon by-passing the thalamus and subthalamus cannot as yet
arouse the direct therapeutic interest of the neurosurgeon, despite
the fact of their functional participation as regards the quality and
extent of painful sensation. On the other hand the remaining fibres
terminating in the various thalamic nuclei may, at present, be
accessible to the surgeon for these reasons. Experimental and clinical experience has conclusively revealed that destruction of only the
main terminal station of pain pathway in the nucleus v.c.pc. is
followed sometimes only by transitional analgesia, at others by only
insufficient hypalgesia and finally sometimes also by the development of hyperpathia. If therefore, we are to eliminate as completely
as possible painful afference and reduce the likelihood of the development of undesirable postoperative states and complications, it becomes advisable to destroy, apart from the "specific" nucleus
n.v.c.pc. (VP), also the neighbouring, in particular the more medially and ventrally located truncothalamic nuclei. This system appar-
ently has a certain antagonistic function towards the spinothalamic
tract and can be released by its isolated destruction.

11. The Pathophysiological Theories of the Central Pain

It is well known that partial interference with the pathways
conducting painful impulses induces generalized impairment of sensitivity and frequently leads to the development of so-called central
pain. In such cases either the first neuron, or the secondary pain

pathway, or finally the thalamic termination might be involved. The causation may be an accident, inflammatory, operative, etc. In these central pains are included mainly causalgia, the postherpetic syndrome, tabetic crises, phantom pain, thalamic pain and anesthesia dolorosa. To this group, however, one must assign also those hyperpathias which originate after therapeutic interventions on the pain pathways in the region of the spinal cord, medulla, mesencephalon or thalamus on account of intractable pain. Whereas such undesirable sequelae form the exception after chordotomy (WHITE and SWEET, 4.3%), their incidence is higher already after transection of the pain pathways in the medulla (CRAWFORD, 8.5%) and still higher following intercollicular mesencephalotomy of WALKER (WALKER, 10%; DRAKE and McKENZIE as much as 50%). Following thalamotomies they are rare too (MONNIER, RIECHERT, COOPER, one own observation).

The development of hyperpathia has not yet been thoroughly elucidated. It is believed to originate as a result of an impaired mutual relationship between myelinated and nonmyelinated afferent fibres. Fibres conducting sensory afference are, as is of course well known, neither structurally nor functionally uniform. Their calibre is diverse with pain conducting fibres either of a large calibre, myelinated and designated as A-delta to epsilon fibres, six to two microns in diameter. These fibres conduct at a rate of up to 20 m./sec. The so-called C-fibres are finer, unmyelinated, of a diameter less than two microns and transmit much more slowly than do the A-fibres, at a velocity of only about 0.6 to 2 m./sec. A-fibres are said to transmit "rapid" pain, C-fibres "slow" pain. Partial interruption of pain conduction also impairs the balance between both groups in favour of fibres conducting more slowly.

HEAD, RIVERS and SHERREN in 1905 already put forward the theory that the pathological qualities of pain sensation originate from irritation of so-called protopathic fibres which, in this functional respect, are identical with the unmyelinated C-fibres (LANDAU and BISHOP) in case of elimination of the second component of sensitivity of the so-called epicritic, identical with transmission by A-fibres. These A-fibres accordingly transmit normal painful impulses which, under ordinary conditions, depress the activity of developmentally lower variants of protopathic sensitivity. DÉJÉRINE and ROUSSY (1906) explain by a similar mechanism of irritation also the development of the thalamic syndrome. HEAD and HOLMES (1912) believed that the thalamic syndrome originates as a result of destruction of corticothalamic tracts exerting a suppressive action. This causes increased thalamic activity and the development of pain. Under ordinary conditions, however, the cerebral cortex controls thalamic activity by means of those tracts. WEDDELL et al. and LIVINGSTON again consider the origin of pathological impulses to be due to reduced innervation density, causing alterations in the quality of pain in the circuit in question. By this mechanism they explain not only the origin of causalgia in peripheral nerve lesions, but also hyperpathia accompanying involvement of the secondary pain pathway, including thalamic pain. Amongst the more recent theories that of SPIEGEL et al. (1953) is worthy of mention. These writers were led to their conclusions by their experiences gained with mesencephalotomies for thalamic pain as well as by experimental studies on cats. Destruction of sensory centres in the thalamus results in transmission of impulses to the hypothalamus, isolation of impulses takes place and pathological impulses for the cortex originate in this way. NOORDENBOS (1959) likewise is a partisan of the theory of the release effect in the slowly transmitting C-fibres in the presence of involvement of the myelinated A-fibres and calls this mechanism "dissociation" of fibres. However, whether we incline more to one or the other theory, all of them show us, or at least suggest, that in neurosurgical practice as regards antalgic operations, also the subsidiary pain conducting pathways should be interrupted, bearing in mind the possibility of hyperpathia.

12. The Blood Supply of the Thalamus

As regards the blood supply of the thalamus, this is realized mainly by branches of the basilar artery. In general, the posterior and ventral region of the thalamus has a more abundant blood supply than the dorsal and anterior region.

Branches of the internal carotid artery, namely the anterior choroid artery supply the dorsolateral thalamic surface, nucleus reticularis thalami and the lateral corpus geniculatum. It is not certain whether this is the terminal vessel. It appears that it at least occasionally forms anastomoses with the posterior cerebral artery. The anteroventral part of the thalamus is also supplied by the so-called striatal arteries arising in the region of the carotid bifurcation. Finally, arteria communicans posterior is the largest carotid branch sharing in the more extensive supply of the thalamus. Its posterolateral branches reach the ventral part of the thalamus and supply the lamina medullaris ventralis, fasciculus mamillothalamicus, nuclei of the massa intermedia and nuclei VA, VPM and VPL.

The main blood supply to the thalamus, however, stems, as already said, from the posterior cerebral artery. Posteromedial branches of the posterior cerebral artery supply the extensive posteroventral part of the thalamus, VPM, VPL and VL. Another branch, the thalamogeniculate artery, whose destruction is most frequently followed by the development of the thalamic syndrome DÉJÉRINE-ROUSSY, emits penetrating small branches also supplying the pulvinar and posterior thalamus. This artery afterwards divides into the thalamic and geniculate arteries. The thalamic artery follows the dorsal surface of the thalamus emitting penetrating branches throughout its course. The geniculate artery supplies pulvinar, lateral geniculate body, habenular region and the pineal gland. Here, surrounding the pineal it creates a fine vascular network from anastomosing branches of the posterior and anterior cerebral arteries.

IV. Surgical Technique

As was already revealed by the historical review of procedures, surgical problems connected with operations on mesencephalon and thalamus are by no means simple. Likewise the ways of approach which stood up to the test of evolution and are used at present for interventions at the various levels of both structures offer some advantages and merits as well as possessing some shortcomings.

Altogether three surgical routes and methods for destruction of pathways conducting pain in the mesencephalon and thalamus exist which fulfill contemporary physiological and clinical requirements demanded of such operations:

1. The open occipital supra-transtentorial approach (WALKER).
2. The open suboccipital infratentorial approach of the present writer.
3. Stereotaxis.

The occipital approach of WALKER may be used only for interventions in the mesencephalon, the open infratentorial route enables operations on the mesencephalon, posterior thalamus and subthalamus and finally stereotaxis allows the performance of destruction in the mesencephalon as well as the thalamus.

1. Walker's Approach to the Mesencephalon

Access to the mesencephalon according to WALKER is obtained from an occipitoparietal craniotomy. The operation is performed under local anaesthesia with the patient lying on his side. The osteocutaneous flap which must extend about 1 cm. below the transverse sinus (Fig. 14) is turned down, as is the dural flap. The head should be tilted downwards, as a result the brain is spontaneously drawn away from the tentorium by its own weight. In order to further simplify access, it is advantageous to perform lumbar puncture during this phase of operation and leave the cerebrospinal fluid to slowly drain away. The incisura tentorii is now approached by cautiously retracting the occipital and posterior portion of the temporal lobe from the tentorium by means of the brain spoon. For this reason bridging veins, parasagittal as well as mainly those which here open into the transverse sinus, must be ligated in the area of the occipital region. Sometimes it proves even necessary to completely interrupt the bundle of Labbé's veins. Partial dissection of the tentorium is performed during the next stage of operation, from the margin of the incisura, thus providing sufficient access to

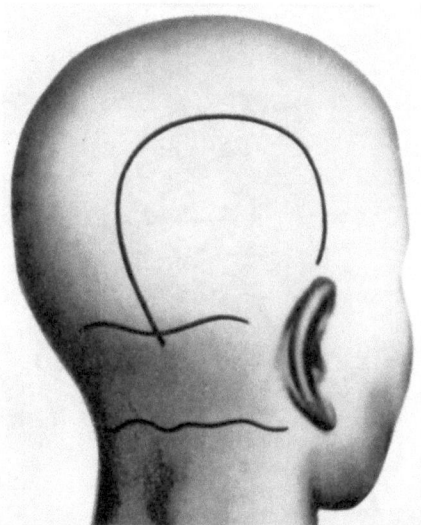

Fig. 14. Skin incision for WALKER's occipital transtentorial approach to the mesencephalon

the region of the cisterna ambiens and quadrigeminal bodies. This approach of WALKER "from above" makes possible the performance of open operations on mesencephalon from its superior colliculi down to the pontomesencephalic juncture. It may thus be used for destruction of pain pathways in mesencephalon, as well as for transection of nigral substance in extrapyramidal disorders. This last opportunity was first exploited by RAND in 1959 (Fig. 15).

WALKER's technique of surgical approach is highly exacting. Its disadvantage lies in the fact that numerous drainage veins in the occipitotemporal region have to be ligated. This interferes with the blood circulation, resulting in congestion and increasing peroperative and postoperative oedema. Dissection of the tentorium, though only partial, is also distressing and time consuming. In order to adhere to the principles of physiological surgery, progress in this location must proceed very slowly, as the tentorium contains a network of venous sinuses which have to be dealt with step by step by suture-ligation, coagulation or clips.

It is not surprising, therefore, that as a result of this route of
approach frequent disturbances of the motor cortex, visual impairment due to ischaemia of the optic radiation and disturbances of
consciousness, as well as complicating haemorrhages (DRAKE and

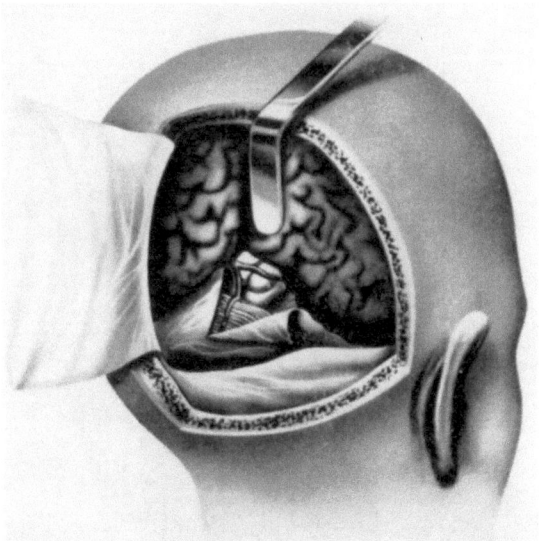

Fig. 15. Approach to mesencephalon by WALKER's occipital route. (For gaining a
better view the occipital lobe is more dislocated than in reality.) Partially from
H. OLIVECRONA and W. TÖNNIS: Handbuch der Neurochirurgie, Bd. 1, 1. Teil,
Grundlagen 1. Berlin-Göttingen-Heidelberg: Springer. 1959

McKENZIE, GLEES and BAILEY), have been reported. This difficult
method of approach makes also a major contribution to the high
mortality rate of WALKER's intercollicular mesencephalic tractotomy, amounting to 23% according to WHITE and SWEET.

2. Guiot's and Forjaz's Modification of the Walker's Operation

GUIOT and FORJAZ proposed a modification of WALKER's occipital approach in the year 1947. In order to avoid ligation of Labbé's
veins and partial dissection of the tentorium, these writers gained
access to the region of corpora quadrigemina more from the front,
by the subtemporal posterior route. However, visualization of the
region of the corpora quadrigemina is not perfect from this approach,
the roof-like prominence of the tentorium is in the way. The danger
of traumatizing important veins draining into the galenic system
and branches of the posterior cerebral and superior cerebellar arteries

is here even greater than when using WALKER's route. This means that this modified technique of GUIOT and FORJAZ did not, in fact, decrease the risk of approach.

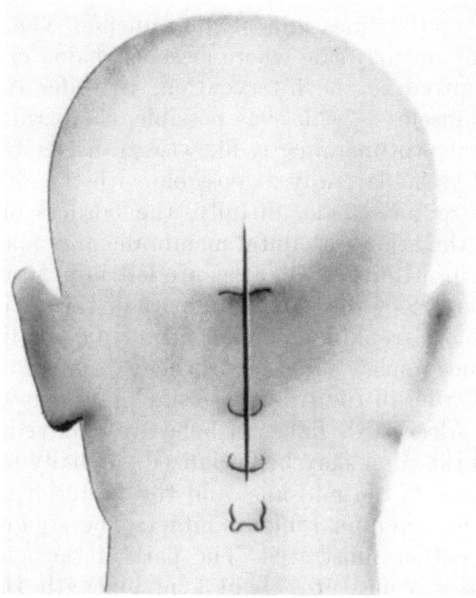

Fig. 16. Skin incision for infratentorial approach to mesencephalon and thalamus

3. The Author's Infratentorial Approach

The operation from the infratentorial suboccipital approach, elaborated by the present writer during the years 1954—1956, may be performed as a one-stage or two-stage procedure. The advantage of the two-stage operation lies in the fact that impairment of sensa tion caused by the operation may be checked during its performance. During the first stage hemicraniectomy of the posterior cranial fossa is done under general endotracheal anaesthesia, the operation proper is done 2—3 days later under local aneasthesia, either in the mesencephalon or thalamus. Both operations are done in the sitting position.

The skin incision is made in the mid-line about 2 cm. above the external occipital protuberance down to the level of the spine of the second cervical vertebra (Fig. 16). Ligamentum nuchae and the subcutaneous layer of connective tissue and fat are divided with the electric scalpel, precisely in the mid-line, in order to avoid unnecessary exposure of the fascial sheaths of the neck muscles. As a rule it is necessary to transect some of the muscle fibres of the rectus capitis posterior at the lower extremity of the incision. Self-retaining retractors are inserted and the periost moved away by raspatory, together with muscular insertions, from the region of the superior and inferior linea and planum nuchae. The occipital bone is exposed only on that side where mesencephalon or thalamus will be later submitted to the intervention. In order to open up the incision and muscles as widely as possible, the periost over the external occipital protuberance is likewise transected longitudinally and dissected as far laterally as possible with the aid of the raspatory. On the required side, distally, the borders of the foramen magnum and the atlantooccipital membrane are exposed, however, the muscular insertions of the atlas are left intact. After obtaining adequate exposure of the squamous part of the occipital bone, at least one or more trephine openings are made, the first preferably close to the linea nuchae superior. During this phase the appearance of the lower border of the transverse sinus must be watched for by direct vision. Afterwards flakes of bone are removed above till the lower third of the sinus may be visualized. Medially bone is chipped away only towards the mid-line, and the posterior osseous border of the foramen magnum remains intact. The squama is chipped away to the extent illustrated. The part of the transverse sinus exposed in this way measures about 3 cm. in length. If the two-stage operation is done, the first phase terminates in suture of the soft tissues by layers (Fig. 17).

If the two-stage operation is done, phase two follows after 2—3 days, this time under local anaesthesia, again in the sitting position. After cutting and removing the sutures, the incision is opened with retractors and the dura mater incised in a halfcircle. The dural incision commences about 5 mm. below the lower border of the transverse sinus. The incision is carried medially under the sinus close to the mid-line, however, damage to the occipital sinus must be avoided. This means that the dura must be opened very cautiously and in small sections, mainly because the sinus need not necessarily be full of blood, particularly in case of cranial hypotension produced orthostatically-due to the sitting position. In such cases sinuses fail to show blue through the dura, they are empty and have the same colour as the neighbouring dura. If the sinus lumen appears during dissection of the dura, it must be immediately compressed with the instrument and sutured, otherwise air embolism from aspirated air might originate, particularly in the case of negative pressure as it was in one of our cases. Laterally the dural incision extends to about 5 mm. from the border of the cut-off bone. The incision is now carried in a downward direction, in a semi-circle, paramedially above the cisterna magna. Thus a small dural flap is produced which is turned over medially. The upper part of the arachnoid fold of the cisterna magna may be seen in the lower medial part of the exposed cerebellar hemisphere.

In order to gain the largest space possible between tentorium and the upper cerebellar surface three to four sutures must be inserted in the upper dural margin beneath the transverse sinus, pulling them taut in a cranial direction. Thus the network of arachnoid trabecules is exposed which, sometimes arranged densely and sometimes more loosely, attach the posterior superior border of the cerebellar hemispheres to the tentorium. These trabecules must be dissected in the exposed segment by elevator under constant visual control in order not to tear some cerebellotentorial bridging veins. These bridging veins, arising from the surface of the quadrangular lobule, are divided, after preceding coagulation, in the space between tentorium and upper cerebellar surface, as they form an obstacle in the route of approach to the cisterna ambiens. Either one or two veins are present, as a rule. Those veins already arising paramedially from the vermis together with those veins running more forward, i.e. the superior vermian vein, supraculminate vein and the precentral cerebellar vein entering the great vein of Galen, are always left intact. By the procedure described so far, sagging of the appropriate cerebellar hemisphere is produced and a space created between its upper surface and the tentorium, sometimes already adequate during this phase for visualizing the arachnoid of the cisterna ambiens. If the space does not appear adequate, slight pressure with the brain spoon may be exerted, however, prior to this it appears advantageous to make a small opening at the upper pole of the exposed part of the cisterna magna, lift up the cerebellar hemisphere and remove the cerebrospinal fluid accumulating from the passages by suction (Figs. 18 and 19).

During the next phase of operation it is frequently necessary to tease away with a fine elevator the anterior paramedial cerebellar margin from arachnoid folds with the ambient cistern. A small opening is made with fine forceps in the arachnoid and extended with the elevator in an upward and mainly in a downward direction parallel with the incisural border of the tentorium.

Immediately in front of the arachnoid there frequently wave about freely in the cistern small branches of the posterior cerebral artery and from the superior cerebellar artery which must not be injured. After disrupting the arachnoid of the cistern part of the tectum with the pineal gland in the mid-line is disclosed above and

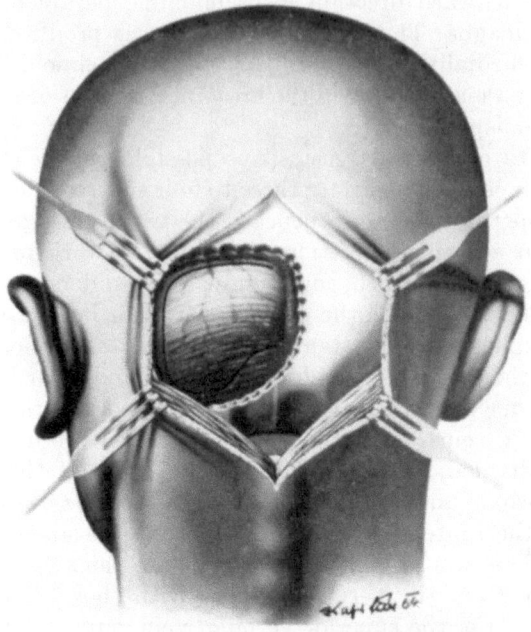

Fig. 17

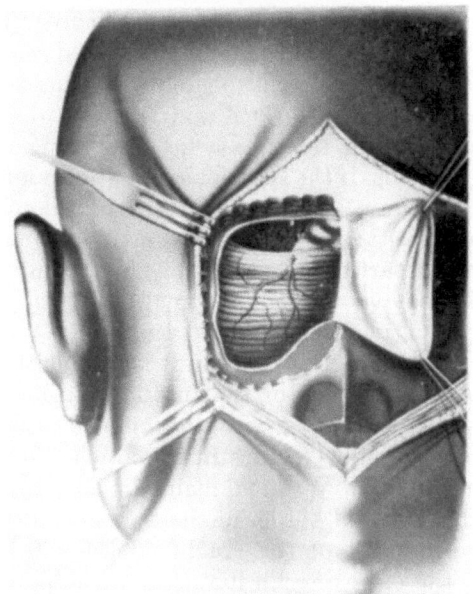

Fig. 18

Figs. 17, 18 and 19. Extent of craniectomy, dural incision ands inking of cerebellar hemisphere with infratentorial approach. (Anteroposterior and lateral projections)

also the colliculus superior with its brachium and the brachium colliculi inferioris. These structures are usually covered with a very fine vascular network, where one can, as a rule, distinctly identify also a small vessel separating both brachia. If WALKER's intercollicular mesencephalotomy is to be performed, the anterior border of

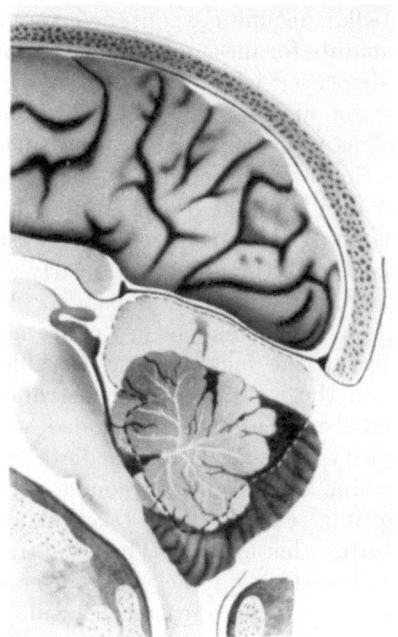

Fig. 19

the cerebellar hemisphere has to be depressed cautiously downwards by means of the brain spoon in order to disclose the lemniscal trigone. The arachnoid of the cisterna ambiens has to be divided as distally as possible for this purpose. The surgical approach to the substantia nigra in cases of extrapyramidal disorders uses an identical procedure. The fine vascular network is drawn aside in the next phase, again using the elevator, but only from the region chosen for the incision. If thalamotomy is to be done the point of juncture between both brachia and c.g.m. is determined and with its immediate neighbourhood stripped off the vascular network. C.g.m. is sometimes already hidden behind the tentorial border. In such cases it becomes necessary to verify the position of the medial border of the c.g.m. by gentle retraction of the tentorial border laterally. This manœuvre must not lead to injury of some neighbouring vessels, i.e. the posterior cerebral artery and the basal vein of Rosenthal closely adjacent to this area.

The infratentorial paramedial approach is advantageous, because no important structures need to be transected, or bruised or retracted. The pressure to which the upper cerebellar surface is exposed by the spoon is only slight. The sagging of the cerebellar hemisphere by itself elicits no transitory functional response. In cases where cerebellar decline is spontaneous and adequate, use of the brain spoon, mainly for mesencephalothalamotomy or for thalamotomy, can be dispensed with. For WALKER's intercollicular mesencephalotomy or for nigrotomy, for which procedures the lateral mesencephalic sulcus represents the guiding surface structure, the frontmost part of the superior cerebellar surface is gently depressed with the spoon. A disadvantage of this approach is the entry of air into the cerebrospinal fluid passages. This results in headache, frequently already during the operation, nearly always after operation, lasting for two, three or more days.

The advantage of the two-stage procedure as against the one-stage operation lies in the fact that we are able in the conscious patient to check on the location of the instrument of destruction by stimulation and also, as already mentioned, we are able to determine, in the majority of cases, the immediate consequences of destruction by checking sensitivity. Of course we are never able to determine the optimal extent of destruction and to predict the lasting result by using this method. The surgical method described is not particularly exacting on the whole, each of the two stages take 30 to 50 minutes. For these reasons, as will be again mentioned in the clinical part of the paper, the intervention may be done in patients already severely affected by chronic and malignant diseases.

Operations in the region of the mesencephalon and thalamus using the open approach may be made more difficult, or even impossible, by vascular variations or anomalies over the quadrigeminal bodies. WALKER mentions already the ectatic venous plexus liable to complicate intervention. It appears that a more abundant venous plexus over the area of the corpora quadrigemina is fairly common, however, as a rule this may be drawn aside from the required section and the operation completed. Out of 70 infratentorial operations on the upper stem done for pain, the present writer encountered only once a compact dilated vascular system, covering the entire posterior incisural region, thus preventing completion of the operation. Apart from this, the mediobasal segment of the hippocampus, overhanging the incisural margin, may interpose itself as an obstacle associated with the infratentorial approach and impeding a clear view of the field of operation. It is advantageous occasionally in such a case to clear away a small part of the overhanging gyrus by cautious suction. From the viewpoint of morbid anatomy such findings, encountered in patients intra vitam, display the pattern of compensated tentorial hippocampal herniation, an entirely insignificant anomaly from the structural and functional angle. This pattern also raises some doubts, as to whether our diagnosis of temporal herniation, seen on the post-mortem table accompanied by the findings of a groove in the hippocampus from the tentorial margin, is always correct.

4. Stereotaxis

Stereotaxis is the third and last method enabling us to destroy even the most distant cerebral structures. Special guiding apparatus is required for this procedure, by means of which the fine instrument for destruction is inserted into the desired area of the brain. The ventricular system must be filled with air or positive contrast medium, in addition, at least one trephine opening must be made and finally an efficient X-ray apparatus must be at one's disposal. From the first construction of stereotactic apparatus for human surgery by SPIEGEL and WYCIS in 1947 a great many simple and more complicated have been manufactured to the date of writing. With their assistance the desired site of the brain should be attained with great precision. This procedure spares structures, often of functional significance, overlying the site of the desired destruction which would be often injured if open approach was used. Tissues are destroyed either mechanically, or by electrolysis, high-frequency coagulation, local freezing, local necrosis through radioactive isotopes, irradiation, or finally selective ultrasonic necrosis. The last mentioned alternative dispenses with the insertion of a probe into the selected site of the brain, however, craniotomy is required for this procedure. With coagulation, the method most commonly used at present, the extent of destruction is, of course, determined by the type, duration and frequency of the current used. It may be relatively easily imagined that the somatotopic arrangement of pain conducting systems in the midbrain and thalamus is less advantageous, than the extrapyramidal centres attacked by this technique in the basal nuclei and stem. Coagulation has to be done repeatedly and in several places in order to achieve satisfactory results in almost every case.

In view of the comparatively complicated arrangement and difficulties of access to these structures, stereotactic destruction of pain

pathways is contemporarily being studied by only a small percentage of workers otherwise engaged in the performance of stereotactic
operations for extrapyramidal disorders. SPIEGEL and WYCIS
possess the greatest experience with the selective destruction of pain
pathways in the midbrain. They were also the first to decide on
performing such operations. ROEDER and ORTHNER, or LEKSELL
found mesencephalotomy satisfactory, whereas RIECHERT, TALAI-
RACH et al., BETTAG and YOSHIDA, MARK and ERVIN and others
express greater hope as regards the control of pain in connection
with operations on thalamic nuclei.

Stereotaxis is an expensive procedure, as stated (RIECHERT),
demanding a perfect technical armamentarium, a team of experts
trained in co-operation and many hours of work. It represents an
advance particularly as regards therapeutico-experimental operations in extrapyramidal disorders. Its use in intractable pain, as
already referred to and as will be the subject of further analysis,
is far less advantageous on account of topographic consideration.

5. Technique of Destructions in the Mesencephalon

The destruction procedure proper is in the operation proposed
by WALKER performed, as a rule, with a straight scalpel, sometimes
also with the electrocoagulation needle, in the mesencephalon. If
one uses the infratentorial approach, it is advisable to perform
WALKER's incision in the midbrain by means of a curved scalpel
with its cutting edge on one side only. Mesencephalothalamotomy,
as will be dealt with later, is done with the same instrument
(Fig. 20).

Now as regards the extent of the incision. In order to achieve
contralateral hemianalgesia of the entire half of the body, the incision must be carried between colliculi, as found by WALKER, from
the lateral sulcus mesencephali across the entire brachium of the
inferior colliculus to the lower border of the superior colliculus. The
incision is 8—10 mm. long (Fig. 5), c. 5 mm. in depth and has an
irregular triangular shape, whose apex extends as far as the lateral
border of the central periaqueductal grey matter. It involves, therefore, the specific spinothalamic tract and, as the case may be, the
bulbothalamic, as well as part of the indirect pain pathways in the
reticular formation of the mesencephalon. Some writers perform the
mesencephalic incision at a somewhat higher level, immediately below the corpus geniculatum mediale (GUIOT and FORJAZ, ZAPLETAL).
This is already on the border of HASSLER's porta thalami, where,
according to anatomical findings, the spinothalamic tract proper is

concentrated into the narrowest calibre. It appears, however, that the reticulothalamic pathways too, terminating in various nuclei of truncothalamic system, are at this juncture between mesencephalon and thalamus more compressed.

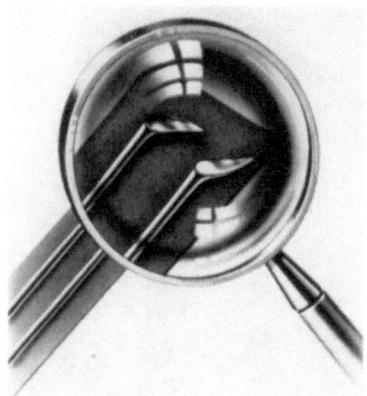

Fig. 20. Curved scalpels with single cutting edge used for mesencephalotomy and mesencephalothalamotomy

6. Technique of the Open Mesencephalothalamotomy

Mesencephalothalamotomy according to the present writer, is best done, as already mentioned, with curved scalpels possessing only one cutting edge, in order to avoid puncturing or transecting the posterior cerebral artery running closely laterally, or injury to branches arising from it, or to important veins. Pain fibres are by this operation destroyed immediately before their entry into the nucleus ventralis parvocellularis (Fig. 21). The scalpel is inserted at the point of juncture brachia-c.g.m. and is carried with its entire cutting edge measuring 7—9 mm. slightly forward and downward towards 6 o'clock. If we wish to eliminate mainly pain fibres for the lower half of the body, we create a sector of the arc by carrying the scalpel laterally towards 3 o'clock on the right or, as the case may be 9 o'clock on the left. Downward the tip of the scalpel should be carried as far as 7 o'clock on the right or, as the case may be, 5 o'clock on the left. If pain arises in the upper half of the body, the sector is created medially again, in the following way. The scalpel is carried as far as 9 o'clock on the dial on the right, or, as the case may be, 3 o'clock on the left. Likewise, the incision is extended still laterally towards 5 o'clock on the right, or 9 o'clock on the left. These incisions also transect the distal part of the nucleus limitans forming part of the truncothalamic system. It is principally that portion of the nucleus called nucleus limitans portae by HASSLER. The nucleus limitans extends furthest laterally and distally out of

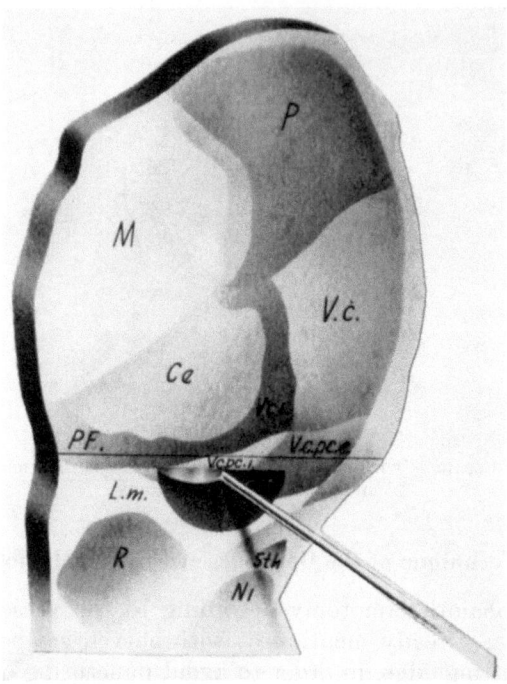

Fig. 21. Cross-section through mesencephalothalamic juncture and extent of destruction during mesencephalothalamotomy for pain in the upper (left) and lower (right) half of the body. The division of nuclei from G. SCHALTENBRAND and P. BAILEY: Introduction to Stereotaxis with an Atlas of the Human Brain. Stuttgart: G. Thieme. 1959

all the truncothalamic system nuclei, almost in front of the whole c.g.m. region. This means that a part of it is destroyed in the course of "medial" as well as "lateral" mesencephalothalamotomy.

7. Stereotactic Destructions

Stereotactic mesencephalotomy or thalamotomy is performed from a frontal, or parietooccipital trephine opening, usually by coagulation needle or cryogenic cannula. As a rule coagulation or freezing must be done repeatedly and in several sites in order to achieve equally extensive destruction, mainly in a mediolateral plane, as in open operations. WYCIS and SPIEGEL have, for these reasons, recently devised a new technique in order to interrupt pain pathways to the greatest extent and certainty. Their procedure is practically likewise already on the borderline between mesencephalon and thalamus, though it is called mesencephalotomy by the writers themselves. SPIEGEL and WYCIS, in patients suffering from pain accompanied by a marked emotional reaction, destroy, apart from the region mentioned, stereotactically also part of the dorsomedial thalamic nucleus. Both these interventions at two different sites are thus called mesencephalothalamotomy by the writers. The present writer, in contrast, as already mentioned, understands by mesencephalothalamotomy transection of afferent pain pathways at the juncture of mesencephalon and thalamus.

LEKSELL also performs stereotactic mesencephalotomy by a similar technique as both American writers. TORVIK, however, was able to detect in two specimens following LEKSELL's mesencephalotomies that stereotactic destruction involved structures in a much larger sector than originally intended. Mainly in the second of the two reported operation cases coagulation involved already more of the thalamus than of the midbrain.

As regards transection of pain conduction systems in the posterior thalamus, the present writer performs them by the open method. Otherwise stereotaxis has so far been used exclusively for these interventions elswhere in the world.

Stereotactic thalamotomy is done from a parietal trephine opening and interrupts as a rule the termination of the specific pain pathway in the n.v.c.pc. (VP) as well as part of the truncothalamic system or also the dorsal region of the posterior thalamus (SPIEGEL-WYCIS and FREE, RIECHERT, MARK and ERVIN). The dorsomedial thalamic nucleus is less frequently included in the destruction with its frontothalamic tracts (SPIEGEL and WYCIS).

8. Technique of Open Thalamotomy

The author performs open thalamotomy by means of the projectable loop-shaped scalpel constructed specially for this purpose. The instrument is constructed on a similar principle as is the leucotome of MONIZ and LIMA, or OBRADOR's cannula, used by this writer for destruction of the globus pallidus in Parkinsonism. The instrument employed by the writer is a little more complicated, delicate and easily controlled. The use of the projectable loop has the advantage of preventing injury to the superficially located structures during penetration towards the desired sector, in this case the corpus geniculatum mediale and the pretectal area. Likewise extent and shape of destruction seems to be more precise, than is the case with other methods.

Details of the loop-shaped scalpel are shown on the drawing attached (Fig. 22 and 23). The scalpel consists of an external

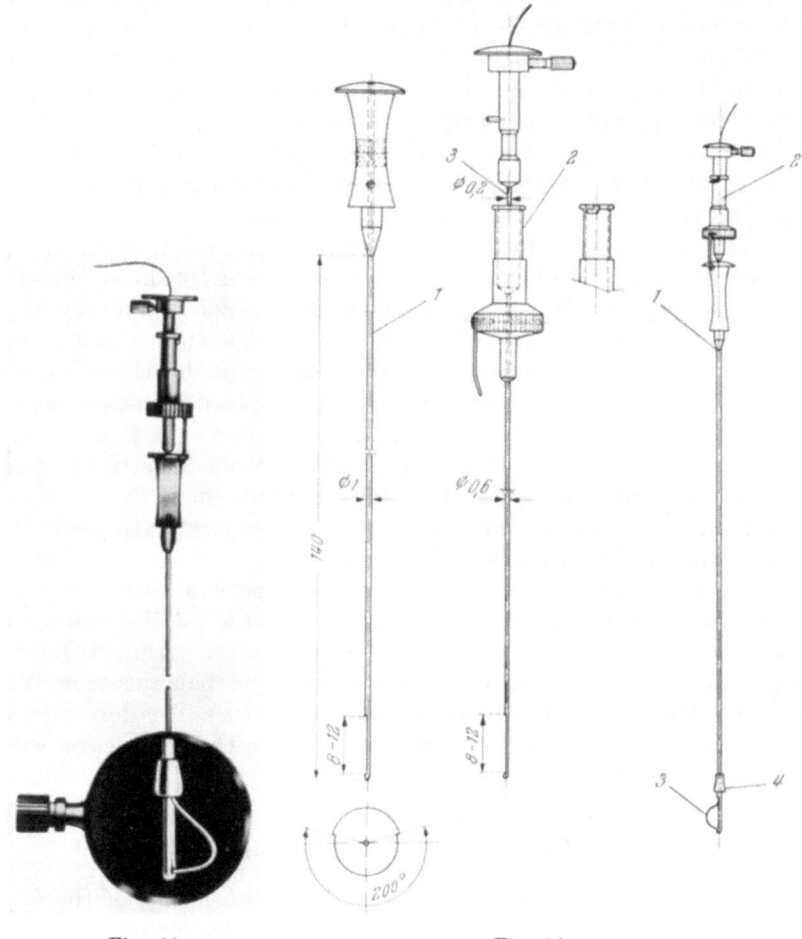

Fig. 22   Fig. 23

Figs. 22 and 23. Detailed views of loop scalpel for open thalamotomy

cannula for insertion (1), an internal cannula (2) and a fine steel wire (3). The external cannula has an outer diameter of 1 mm., the internal of 0,7 mm. The length of the cannula is 140 mm., its tip is rounded. About 1 mm. below the tip is a rectangular opening, encompassing half of the calibre of the cannula, 11 mm. long. The cannula terminates in a rectangular handle measuring 4 mm × 4 mm. about 17 mm. in length. An internal cannula is inserted into the external cannula and it carries an identical rectangular opening near the tip. This internal cannula terminates in a handle measuring about 25 mm. in length. The handle consists of a grooved part with

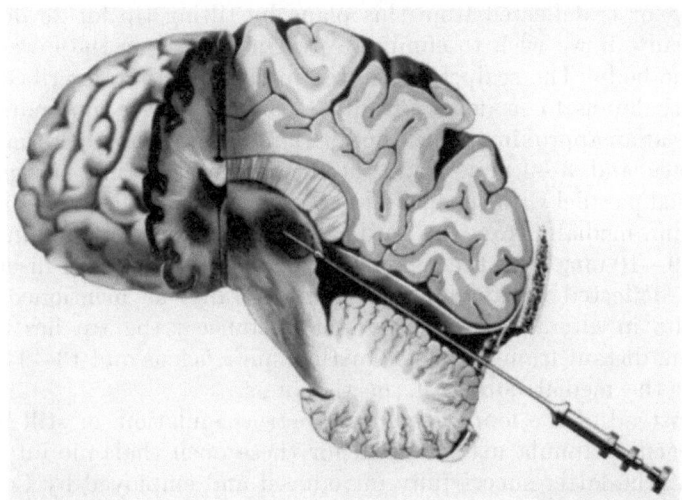

Fig. 24. The open infratentorial thalamotomy with the loop scalpel in situ

an indicator on its outer circumference for limiting rotation of the loop and further out of a bayonet lock for securing and fixing the loop. The loop itself is created by extruding the steel wire measuring 0,2 mm. in diameter. The extruded loop is fixed in the bayonet lock. A small locking device slides along the outer cannula (4).

For actual use of the scalpel, after insertion, the left hand grips the tetragonal handle of the outer cannula, the right hand the wire pusher which is inserted into the bayonet fitting. Thus a loop is created whose size depends, as already mentioned, on the length of the rectangular openings cut in the cannula side and also from the distance adjustment between the small peg from the bayonet fixing the wire by a grooved screw. An X-ray is taken after creation of the loop. Afterwards the grooved part of the internal cannula is gripped by the right hand. By its rotation destruction is now performed. The shape of the loop creates by its rotation to the right and to the left an ovoid destruction. The system of two cannulas has been introduced so that the external cannula may be gripped firmly in the hand and rotation here avoided (Fig. 24).

The tip of the loop scalpel is placed on the landmark c.g.m.-brachia at about 11 to 13 mm. distance from the midline. The tip of the scalpel is deflected caudally by about 45 degrees from the plane carried through the axis of the course of the medulla and distal brain stem. It is inserted either parallel with the medial plane, if we wish to achieve hemianalgesia of mainly the upper part of the body, or is deflected from this plane by tilting tip for 20 degrees laterally, if we wish to eliminate pain mainly from the lower half of the body. The scalpel is inserted in the direction described into the thalamus for a depth of only 12 mm. from the landmark. Its tip is at an approximate distance of 12 mm. from the upper thalamic surface and 3—4 mm. from the thalamosubthalamic margin. If carried parallel with the medial plane, then the needle tip lies about 12 mm. medially from the border of the reticular thalamic nucleus and 9—10 mm. from the medial thalamic border. If, before insertion, it is deflected by about 20 degrees laterally, as mentioned, this results in alterations of individual distances: the tip lies about 7 mm. distant from the reticular thalamic nucleus and 13—14 mm. from the medial border of the thalamus.

Instead of the loop scalpel an electrocoagulation, or still better cryogenic cannula may be used for these open thalamic interventions, the latter successfully introduced and employed by COOPER and others, by FUSEK in my country. In my view the freezing cannula offers an advantage not possessed by any other method of destruction of deep cerebral structures by producing sharply demarcated lesions (COOPER), without danger of extensive haemorrhage in the neighbourhood of destruction. A disadvantage of stereotactic operation remain in this respect the channels of insertion made through the entire transversal or oblique cross section of the thalamus in operations for pain.

The radius of the released loop now used by us as standard procedure is 6.5—7 mm., which means that the diameter of destruction ovoid in shape amounts to 12—14 mm. This is a larger lesion than set e.g. by COOPER. His destructions measure only 3—10 mm. Another difference lies in the fact, that the location of lesions made by the open approach consists of one selective insertion aimed at the region for either the upper or lower part of the body, as already described, and does not aim in particular at involving other structures such as the central nucleus of the thalamus etc., likewise it does not alter its course in a craniocaudal direction.

9. The Extent of Thalamic Destructions.
The "Partial Longitudinal Thalamotomy"

The object of these interventions in the thalamus is the destruction of the major part of the ventrocaudal nucleus and part of the truncothalamic system with medial subthalamic area. By penetra-

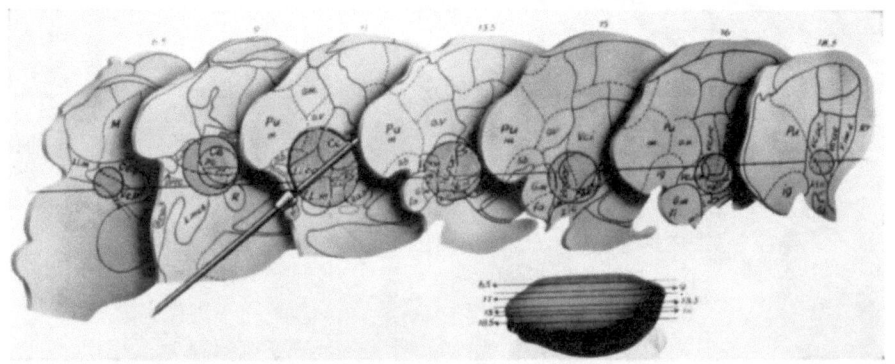

Fig. 25. Extent of destruction of ventrocaudal nucleus and intrathalamic nuclei by loop scalpel in seven sagittal sections. The division of thalamic nuclei from G. SCHALTENBRAND and P. BAILEY: Introduction to Stereotaxis with an Atlas of the Human Brain. Stuttgart: G. Thieme. 1959

tion of the scalpel loop to a depth of 12 mm. from the juncture c.g.m.-brachia, mainly part of the central nucleus or nucleus parafascicularis are destroyed and also a small proportion of frontothalamic fibres entering the medial nuclei (Fig. 25). Our clinical experiences revealed that this small destruction has no effect whatsoever on either personality of the patient, or pain reactivity and also fails to produce any frontal symptomatology. We were, however, able to observe that destruction of a still larger number of fibres of the tracts mentioned caused by penetration by the scalpel with extruded loop pointing dorsally, further to the front, results in progressively more marked mental disturbances which, even with unilateral operation, may produce persistent and identical patterns, as we are already acquainted with from bilateral lobotomy in the frontal lobes. If part of these tracts is interrupted at a distance of 18—19 mm. from the point of juncture c.g.m.-brachia, i.e. approximately the posterior half of the thalamus, pain reactivity is altered as a result of such an intervention, the patient sometimes experiencing even slight euphoria, otherwise, however, none of the undesirable personality changes as well as mental defects with gatism etc. are produced by it, as may be observed after destruction of the medial thalamic nucleus, or after frontal operations. For these reasons, the operation described, named "partial longitudinal thalamotomy," is recommended mainly for central pain, or in cases

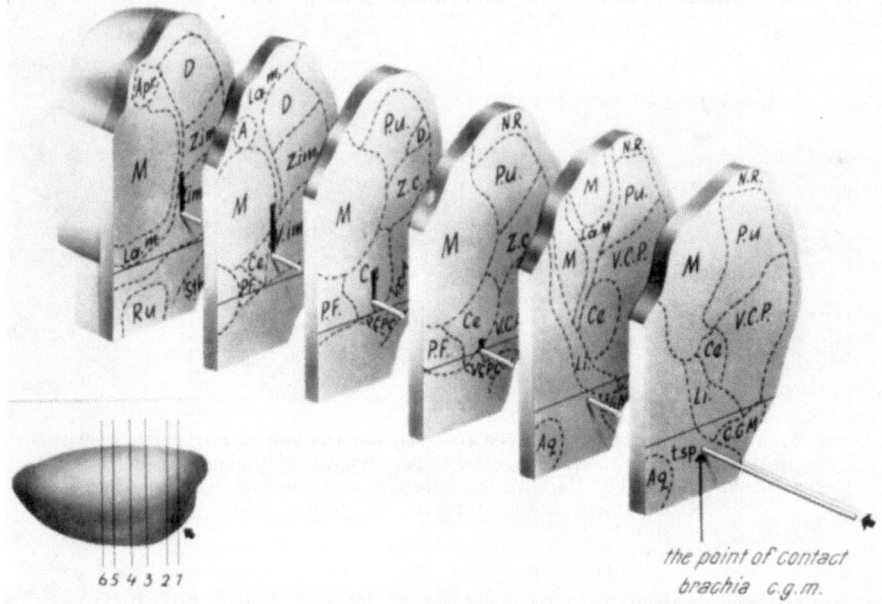

Fig. 26. Extent and localization of thalamic destruction for partial longitudinal thalamotomy in six transverse sections. The division of thalamic nuclei from G. SCHALTENBRAND and P. BAILEY: Introduction to Stereotaxis with an Atlas of the Human Brain. Stuttgart: G. Thieme. 1959

where a marked affective component of pain governs the picture. It is performed in cases, where SPIEGEL and WYCIS at present recommended partial destruction of the dorsomedial nucleus of the thalamus, or WHITE modified unilateral frontal lobotomy (Fig. 26).

The extruded loop, pointing consistently vertically upward, must not, of course, be rotated in performing partial longitudinal thalamotomy. At the distance of approximately 18 mm. from c.g.m., as described, there lies the nucleus ventralis intermedius somewhat laterally, the terminus of dentatorubrothalamic and striothalamic fibres. These were interfered with in one of our patients, when rotation of the scalpel after preceding longitudinal thalamotomy was done too much in front.

10. Side-effects and Complications of Mesencephalotomies and Thalamotomies

Obviously, destruction of pain pathways in the mesencephalon or thalamus, whether performed by the open method or by stereotaxis, is accompanied by simultaneous interruption of other nervous systems and tracts, some of whom play an important functional role. In the classical incision of WALKER the brachium colliculi inferioris is transected with the secondary acoustic pathway in the lateral lemniscus, as well as part of the medial lemniscus with sensory afferents and part of the reticular formation of the tegmentum, sometimes also with a small section of the central periaqueductal grey matter. Incisions performed at the level of the colliculus superior and in mesencephalothalamotomy, are less frequently accompanied by damage to the lateral lemniscus, the same applies to c.g.m. whose medial portion is injured as a rule. These interventions also involve a part of the nucleus limitans, particularly that part called limitans portae by HASSLER. This is of course, in the light of contemporary knowledge of the physiology of pain conduction, a highly desirable effect. Upper mesencephalotomy after SPIEGEL and WYCIS is sometimes accompanied by injury to a major portion of the centre for pupillary reflexes, area pretectalis. Destruction of thalamic nuclei may result in the origin of psychic disturbances, mainly in cases of injury to a major part of the medial nucleus, or its frontothalamic and thalamofrontal fibres. This may happen accidentally in planned destruction of the medial nucleus (SPIEGEL and WYCIS), or with the partial longitudinal thalamotomy of the writer. The occasionally seen impairment of taxis and cerebellar disturbances of gait, persisting as a rule for a short period only, are caused by lesions of the nucleus ruber, of rubrothalamic fibres or, as the case may be, direct or indirect lesion of the ventral intermedial thalamic nucleus located in front of the ventrocaudal nucleus. A similar pattern may originate also following excessively extensive thalamic destruction possibly inducing the development of the thalamic syndrome. This was described by RIECHERT, however, its origin was ascribed to unduly small destruction. We were ourselves able to observe the development of the thalamic syndrome in a patient operated elsewhere: R. A., aged 40 years suffering from severe phantom syndrome. In 1960 he had a motorcycling accident accompanied by avulsion of the brachial plexus on the left and his left subclavian artery was torn and bruised. The vessel was sutured, however, a fortnight later severe suppuration originated in the paralysed limb associated with general sepsis. His left arm had to be

amputated above the elbow. Severe phantom pains started one
month after amputation relieved only by opiates. Neither procain
infiltrations nor psychotherapy had any effect. Accordingly two
stage destruction of v. c. and surroundings was performed. The patient was entirely symptom free for a fortnight after operation,
however, phantom sensation started to reappear and after 4 months
also pains of a pricking character in the stump and only a little better
tolerated than before operation. From this time onwards the patient
demanded opiates with vigour. A proposal for sleep therapy was
turned down by him. There was objective evidence of persisting
complete analgesia of the upper half of the body with tactile hyper-
pathy in the region of the amputation stump and shoulder. The
patient was six months after our operation submitted to stereotactic destruction of the medial nucleus at another centre, according
to a report. Three weeks after this intervention severe pain and
"pins and needles" developed in the left foot, chilling sensations
in the left side of the face, chest and hip. These symptoms proved
so intolerable and were not relieved even by high doses of morphia,
that the patient, as reported by his family, committed suicide
shortly afterwards.

    However, luckily, thalamic pains after destruction of thalamic
nuclei for pain originate only very exceptionally (MONNIER; RIE-
CHERT; BETTAG and YOSHIDA: COOPER). If we take into account,
on the other hand, the excellent effect of thalamotomy in cases of
the thalamic syndrome Déjérine-Roussy, as demonstrated by TA-
LAIRACH et al., our existing pathophysiological shortcomings are
brought into still more striking relief. It appears that the action
mechanism in this case also will be similar as in pallidum destruction, destruction of the ventrooral nucleus of the thalamus, the substantia nigra or the subthalamic region in parkinsonism, accompanied, as known, also by the most pronounced structural changes
particularly in the substantia nigra and pallidum.

11. Stimulation of Pain Pathways at the Brain Stem Levels

    Stimulation of pain pathways and nuclei respectively by high
frequency alternating current was done in numerous patients before
destruction. This was done by me mainly in mesencephalotomies,
during that first phase of operations on the stem during which I
destroyed only segmental sections of painful afferents. Stimulation
of pain fibres in the mesencephalon and the mesencephalothalamic
juncture in the porta thalami always resulted in sharp limited pain
in the corresponding body regions. Sometimes pain was felt in a

larger area of the contralateral half, sometimes in the entire half of the body. Stimulation of thalamic nuclei sometimes caused sharp and precisely localized pain, but sometimes patients stated to experience only diffuse, burning and highly unpleasant sensations, to which they frequently reacted by rapid defensive movements of the extremities and groaning.

Stimulation of pain pathways and nuclei preceding destruction proper is of value particularly with stereotactic operations, where it determines the correct location of the probe (UMBACH, 1966). In open operations, as performed by the writer, this manœuvre is necessary only in segmental destructions. These, however, were found to be indicated, in view of their transitory effect, only in patients whose survival period was assumed to be short.

12. Anatomical and Histological Findings

As regards the further procedure in infratentorial operation: after destruction has been completed, the loop of the scalpel is withdrawn and the instrument pulled out. So far we have never observed any haemorrhage from the needle opening after its withdrawal. However, if we have failed to clear the vascular network from the surface thoroughly, a small subarachnoid collection of blood develops sometimes in this site. In such cases we cover denuded surface of the quadrigeminal bodies with a small piece of fibrin foam. The dura is sutured meticulously after that, as are the remaining soft tissues by layers.

Necropsy findings in persons submitted to infratentorial operations on the stem, reveal that this approach causes no gross changes. The sole abnormality found, as a rule, is the damaged arachnoid at the juncture of posterior and superior cerebellar surfaces due to blunt dissection of the network of arachnoid trabecules, and also in the places where veins had to be coagulated.

As shown on the appended photographs of the brain specimens (Figs. 27 and 28) from two patients who underwent thalamotomy and died at the end of the operation from air embolism (pat. No. 39) and on the 10th post-operative day from pneumonia (pat. No. 42), the site for destruction may be selected with great precision. Likewise the extent of the lesion is relatively small, but operation on patient No. 42 achieved skin analgesia with complete relief from pain.

Experiences gained so far reveal that we are able to achieve analgesia of the appropriate part of the body and thereby also lasting relief from somatic pain by performing destruction in the mesencephalon, on the mesencephalothalamic juncture, or in the thalamus. In WALKER's or the present writer's open operation, structures selected for destruction are located immediately below the surface of the denuded stem. The position of thalamic nuclei, nucleus limitans, nucleus centralis thalami with nucleus parafascicularis, nucleus

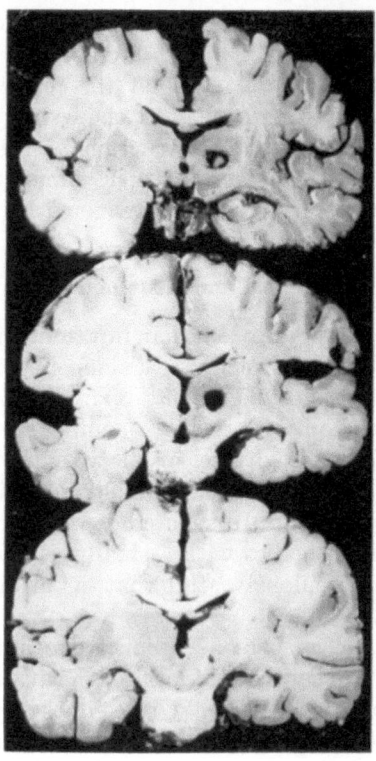

Fig. 27. Extent of thalamic destruction in three brain sections (Pat. No. 39). Elaborated by J. Dušek, M.D., from the Institute of Pathological Anatomy, Olomouc

ventrocaudalis parvocellularis and the zona incerta of the subthalamus, is particularly advantageous for antalgic operations by the open route, as already stated. The superficial position of these structures guarantees, that the destruction can be done with great precision and under visual control. In stereotaxis the target of the instrument for destruction is located at some distance and invisible. Already for these reasons stimulation should be done before destruction in order to determine the exact position of the probe. Not only the terminal stations of pain pathways may be destroyed if the infratentorial approach is used, but interruption of the fronto-thalamic and thalamofrontal tracts may also be performed by the so-called partial longitudinal thalamotomy. It is quite certain that

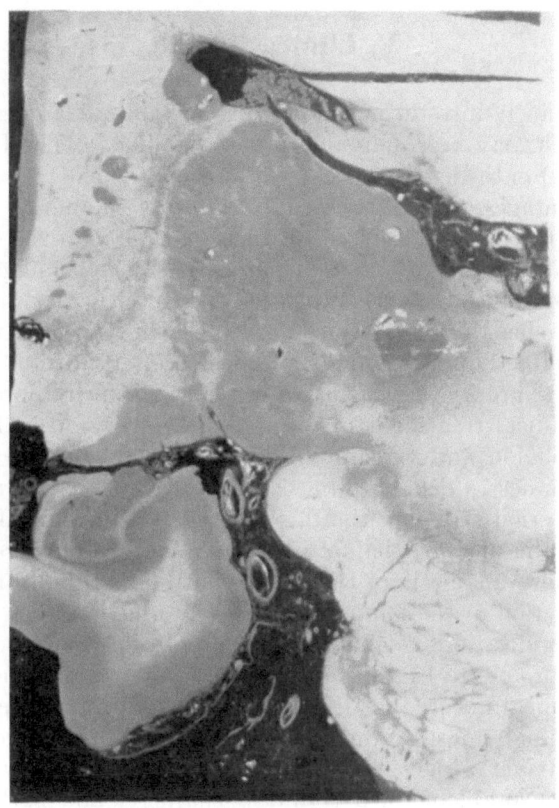

Fig. 28. Extent of thalamic destruction on the histotopogram (Pat. No. 42), Elaborated by J. Dušek, M.D., from the Institute of Pathological Anatomy, Olomouc

selection of any of the available operations will depend on the personal experiences of the surgeon who will select amongst the various methods the one he has become familiar with, simplified and perfected its technique and which he will prefer for the reasons stated. The topographic arrangement of systems in mesencephalon and thalamus for conducting pain, however, in the writer's opinion, offers more reliable results with the open method.

V. Clinical Results

Each newly introduced therapeutic method undergoes its evolution which may be subdivided into three phases. The first is as a rule full of enthusiasm and associated with the endeavour to stress the advantages and advance contributed by the newly introduced method. In contrast, the second phase is characterized by various degrees of depression emanating from the shortcomings and risk accompanying the new therapeutic procedure. A certain balance is finally reached during the third phase, when it is possible to evaluate the whole method after an adequate time interval from its "birth" using an appropriate measure of critical and open approach.

The radical treatment of intractable pain by operations in the mesencephalon and thalamus also underwent such an evolution, and continues to develop in accordance with the rules mentioned. After a period stressing the fact that transection of afferent pain tracts in the mesencephalon, or destruction of appropriate nuclei, may achieve analgesia of the entire contralateral half of the body, dissatisfaction arose comparatively early and was due to the frequent complications, mainly in the field of hyperpathia. This phase was also prolonged by the considerable complications and obstacles of a technical nature, as already referred to in preceding chapters. The terminal phase of final evaluation and critical review thus remains as yet widely open and delayed by still relatively limited experience, problems of a technical character and pathophysiological problems. It was also the writer's object to contribute to the solution of some points of the still open problems of mesencephalotomy and thalamotomy and thereby also to the evaluation and estimation of the utility of these methods. It appears, however, that antalgic operations in the mesencephalon and at the junction of mesencephalon and thalamus have been abandoned to-day with a few exceptions and that destruction of thalamic nuclei has been accepted as the best method for all operations on the brain stem and medulla.

1. Indications for the Brain Stem Operations and the Division of Patients for the Resultant Evaluation

Operations of the midbrain and thalamus were advised in all patients suffering from persistent pain, refractory to other methods of treatment. If pain was due to neoplastic conditions, the general health of the patient had to be such as to offer a prognostic hope of several weeks survival. Patients suffering from marked cardiovascular or pulmonary disorders, with severe cachexia or serious mental disturbances were not accepted for operation. Slight myocardial changes, arteriosclerosis, unilateral pleural effusion, or minor degrees of cachexia did not contraindicate operation.

The writer, during the years 1955—1965, performed a total of 70 operations in the mesencephalon and thalamus for intractable pain affecting 51 patients. Detailed data on pain localization and individual operations are listed in Table 1. This reveals that about

Table 1. *Total number and localization of operations in the mesencephalon and thalamus*

Site of pain	Mesencephalotomy	Mesencephalothalamotomy	Thalamotomy (n.v.c.pc.)	Destruction of nucleus dorsomedialis thalami	Partial longitudinal thalamotomy	Combination with contralateral chordotomy
Head			1			
Upper limbs, Neck, Thorax	10	4	13		6	
Abdomen, Pelvis	12	9	7	2	1	9
Lower limbs	2	1				
Total number	24	14 (+ 2 reoperations)	21	2	7	9

half the operations were done for pain in the abdomen and pelvis or lower extremities respectively. The writer decided to perform these operations also in cases of pain in the lower parts of the body for a variety of reasons. In the first place he is convinced that the infratentorial technique of approach is no more exacting for the patient than is laminectomy for chordotomy, though, of course, this does not apply in relation to the surgeon. Secondly, these operations were performed in cases of carcinoma of the rectum and uterus, because pain localized in the mid-line of the sacral segments is not easily influenced by chordotomy (WHITE and SWEET). In these conditions and in bilateral pain, either bilateral mesencephalotomy was tried, or operations on the mesencephalon and thalamus respectively in combination with contralateral chordotomy. Finally it was the writer's aim to ascertain the usefulness of segmental operations. As may be seen from the topographic description, pain pathways for the lower half of the body are particularly suitably located for this purpose. Otherwise the writer chose operations on the upper thoracic spinal cord during the period under review only in cases of isolated pain affecting one lower extremity, eventually a medial longitudinal myelotomy in cases of pain affecting both lower extremities.

In nine women one of the described interventions on the stem was done for metastases of breast cancer. The women concerned were mainly suffering from intolerable pain in the upper extremity due to compression of lymphatic and venous drainage by metastases or due to direct involvement of the brachial plexus. In the remaining patients with breast cancer metastases either hypophysectomy is done, or these patients are treated by adrenalectomy.

For the evaluation of the results of operation 4 grades of assessment will be used in all cases. The first grade signifies disappearance or substantial relief from pain to such a degree that it becomes possible to discontinue the administration of opiates, other analgetics or sedative drugs. Complications in respect of hyperpathia are absent in this group, only indifferent sensation in the desafferented part of the body. Second grade signifies reduction of pain by 30—50%, or the original pain disappears completely, however, dysaesthesias develop which are weaker than the original pain. In grade three the condition of the patient remains unchanged, or hyperpathias develop troubling the patient as much as the preoperative pain. Finally in grade four pain and general symptoms deteriorate after operation, most frequently as a result of severe hyperpathia developing, or due to other serious complications. The result of operation is evaluated in each case according to these criteria firstly during the postoperative phase, amounting to 8 weeks, and secondly during the phase following this 8 week interval and called the late phase.

The period of 8 weeks is certainly quite inadequate for verification of the lasting effect of operation. It was selected despite its shortness in view of the fact that the majority of patients suffering from neoplastic disease survived for only a few weeks or months. We know that the likelihood of long-term persistence in antalgic operations on the spinothalamic tract and its termination in the thalamus is determined in the first place by the extent of algic skin disturbances (WHITE and SWEET; RIECHERT). Likewise our results

confirm that a return to normal of the hypalgesia setting in already
a few days after operation means that relief from organic pain
exceeding a period of 1—3 weeks may not be expected. It seems
likely, therefore, that the patients of MARK and ERVIN who failed
to experience any impairment of sensitivity, but were satisfactorily
relieved of pain, achieved this result only in view of their short
survival.

As regards clinical results of interventions in the mesencephalon,
it appears preferable to evaluate these according to results of open
operation, called mesencephalic tractotomy by some writers, than
according to stereotactic interventions, designated as mesencephalotomy. However, some other writers use the term mesencephalotomy
also for open operations. In the latter it is possible, as already
mentioned, to place and determine the extent of the incision more
precisely than by stereotaxis. The position and topography of the
mesencephalon are very disadvantageous for stereotaxis, as also
admitted by SPIEGEL and WYCIS who have recently been trying to
perfect their technique by alteration in the direction of the needle.
A majority of stereotactic operations in the upper mesencephalon
lead to much more extensive destruction than is as a rule performed
during open operations, frequently also affecting the region of the
thalamus, in reality, constituting extensive mesencephalothalamotomies, as shown by TORVIK. For these differences in principle,
results of open operations and results of stereotactic interventions
will be submitted to separate analysis.

2. The Classical Walker's Operation

The pioneer of antalgic operations on the mesencephalon EARL
WALKER performed 13 mesencephalotomies by the open route, with
a single postoperative death. This writer reported in detail on the
first five cases. By his classical intercollicular incision he achieved
contralateral hemianalgesia of the entire half of the body, including
the face. Hemianalgesia sometimes changed into hypalgesia with
gradual recovery. In metastatic pain with a short period of survival
WALKER was able to observe satisfactory relief, in central pain he
saw only temporary improvement. Troublesome hyperpathias
developed in 10% cases. As a direct result of the approach route
WALKER described the development of hemianopsia in two cases.
However, DRAKE and McKENZIE, though achieving perfect analgesia in five out of six cases by the intercollicular incision, this was
later followed in three i.e. 50% by severe hyperpathias. In two of
these six cases perception for high tones was reduced, as shown by

audiography. In five of these cases there also arose temporary, but complete hemianopsia due to a lesion of the occipital lobe. Results of other writers with the classical operation of WALKER in the mesencephalon are also similar (WHITE and SWEET; SJÖQVIST; BAILEY; ZAPLETAL). BAILEY and GLEES and coworkers performed a small number of mesencephalotomies using WALKER's open route, observed their patients in detail clinically and also made anatomical studies. They determined the accurate location of ascending and descending pathways in the dorsolateral portion of the mesencephalon, the site for incision, by studying degeneration of fibres. The writers saw in a female patient whose case they reported and analysed in their paper published in 1954, transitory somnolence and incontinence as well as permanent phatic disturbances following intercollicular mesencephalotomy with an incision of 8 mm × 4 mm. on the left. The patient lost her pain up to her death which took place 4 months later and suffered only slight dysaesthesias which did not trouble her. The writers conclude from their experience that mesencephalic tractotomy is a major operation, but that it is safer than medullary tractotomy. Antalgic destruction in the mesencephalon affects numerous afferent paths, such as the medial lemniscus, lateral spinothalamic tract, quintothalamic tract, lateral lemniscus and other ascending pathways; amongst descending tracts mainly the tractus tegmentoolivaris whose transection appears to have no perceptible functional consequences.

In summary, WALKER's intercollicular incision serves to achieve analgesia of the contralateral half of the body and a very good antalgic effect, however, in a high percentage cases are afflicted by the development of hyperpathia and very frequently also by audiographic changes, sometimes accompanied by subjective impairment of hearing. Marked disorders of hearing bordering on deafness originate after bilateral mesencephalotomy of WALKER (WALKER; MIKULA, ŠIROKÝ and ZAPLETAL). As a consequence of using the occipital route of approach, hemianopsia develops frequently, as also do paresis and phatic disturbances, exceptionally also disturbances of consciousness (BAILEY-GLEES and OPPENHEIMER).

WALKER already attempted to avoid the above mentioned serious complications of the intercollicular mesencephalic incision, mainly the impairment of hearing, by transection of only part of the painful afference. He based this step mainly on his own experimental results showing that fibres conducting pain have a segmental distribution also in the mesencephalon. GUIOT and FORJAZ attempted segmental transection of pathways in one patient. They transected part of the pain pathways a little above the classical incision of

WALKER with the object of eliminating pain in the upper part of the body on account of phantom pain of the thumb in the upper limb. After the incision, conducted in a medioventral direction, they observed a painless interval of 2 months duration accompained by gradually recovering hemihypalgesia.

3. The Author's Clinical Results with Mesencephalotomy

As shown on Table 2, the writer performed—during the years 1955 to 1957—a total of 24 open operations in the mesencephalon on 18 patients. Five patients had bilateral segmental operation, in one case mesencephalic operation had to be repeated as the first operation failed to provide sufficient relief and in another two mesencephalothalamotomy was done after mesencephalotomy had failed. These patients are the first two cases in the list of mesencephalothalamotomies figuring in Table 3.

There were 10 females and 8 males amongst the 18 patients (Table 2). Fourteen were suffering from pain due to neoplastic disease. There were five cases of breast cancer metastases, two cases of metastatic uterine cancer, three cases of cancer of the rectum with metastases, one patient had carcinoma of the larynx, one fibrosarcoma of the neck, another sarcoma of the soft tissues of the arm and finally the last had retroperitoneal malignancy. Another female patient from this group of mesencephalotomies had causalgic pain of the hand following amputation of a finger, one male had phantom pains in the lower limb, two patients were suffering from tabetic crises. The oldest patient operated was a female aged 67 years with tabetic anorectal crises, the youngest a female aged 25 with sarcoma of the neck.

Out of these 18 patients one male aged 65 years with recurrence of laryngeal carcinoma died on the fifth postoperative day from severe bilateral bronchopneumonia. Segmental incision measuring 6 mm. × 5 mm. achieved hemianalgesia of the upper half of the body with hypalgesia of the lower half and disappearance of pain. In view of the fact that this patient died during the early postoperative phase he will be excluded from further evaluation of results. The postoperative course was uneventful in the remaining patients and intervention itself never caused any serious complications. In one female aged 34 years with metastatic breast cancer (No. 3) tracheotomy had to be done on account of postoperative oedema of the vocal cords for a period of 4 days. Another patient (No. 18), who had a bilateral operation for tabetic gastric crises, had uncontrollable hiccup three days after operation disappearing spontaneously on the fourth day.

Table 2. *Mesencephalotomy*

No.	Name, Age, Sex	Basic disease	Operation (Extent of incision, length × depth)	Operat. result immed. 1	2	3	4	late 1	2	3	4	Damage of algic sensation	Complications	Notes
1	E. V. 55, w.	Ca. mammae dx.	9 × 5 mm. sec. WALKER sin.		+							analgesia dx.	mild hyperpathias, reduct. of tactile sens., kinesthes.	corneal reflex reduced. died 4 weeks later
2	E. A. 52, w.	Ca. mammae dx.	6 × 4 mm. segm. sin.		+				+			hypalges. more in lower parts dx.	mild hyperpathias	ectatic veins over quadrigeminal bodies
3	L. M. 34, w.	Ca. mammae dx.	6 × 5 mm. segm. sin.			+					+	mild hypalges. dx.	severe hyperpathias, tracheostomy, tactile hypaesthesia	
4	M. K. 66, w.	Ca. mammae sin.	6 × 8 mm. segm. dx.			+					+	marked hypalges. sin. dx.	severe hyperpath., 3 days tinnitus, depression	died 7 months later
5	J. P. 33, w.	Ca. mammae dx.	4 × 4 mm. dx. 4 × 4 mm. s. segm., medial.	+				+				diminishing hypalges. Th 2—S 5	numbness in the right leg	died 3 months later
6	V. F. 34, w.	Ca. uteri	5 × 4 mm. dx. 5 × 4 mm. s. segm., later.		+				+			hypalges. Th 12—S 5	mild hyperpathias, tinnitus bil. more on left	loss of preoperative anorexia, died 4 months later
7	M. B. 42, w.	Ca. uteri	5 × 3 mm. dx. 6 × 5 mm. s.	+				+				marked hypalges. dx. (sin.: 0)	temporary tinnitus, more dx.	died 10 weeks later

Table 2 (continuation)

No.	Name, Age, Sex	Basic disease	Operation (Extent of incision, length × depth)	Operat. result immed. 1	2	3	4	late 1	2	3	4	Damage of algic sensation	Complications	Notes
8	K. B. 39, m.	Ca. recti	3 × 5—6 mm. sin., segm., later.	+			+				+	mild hypalges. Th 12—S 5 dx.	marked hyperpath. in the right lower limb	refused reoperation
9	F. K. 54, m.	Ca. recti	5 × 5 mm. dx. segm., later.			+				+		analgesia Th 12—S 5 sin.	excruciating anal pain unrelieved	mesencephalothalamotomy 4 weeks later
10a	F. P. 46, m.	Ca. recti	2 × 5 mm. s. segm., later.	+		+						analgesia sin.		two days later mesencephalothalamotomy died the 5th day post operat. of bilateral bronchopneumonia
11	V. S. 65, m.	Ca. laryngis	6 × 5 mm. dx.	+								analgesia sin.		died 2 months later
12	M. R. 25, w.	Sa. colli dx.	6 × 5 mm. dx.	+						+		hypalges. sin.	hyperpathias slight reduction of tactile sensation	
13	J. B. 47, m.	Sa. humeri sin.	6 × 5 mm. dx.			+				+		analgesia upper limb, hypalges. lower limb	hyperpathias, tinnitus, tactile sensib. reduced	
14	J. P. 60, m.	Teratoma retro-periton.	6 × 6 mm. s. segm., later.	+					+			analgesia L 1—S 5 dx.		sensation was affected already before, therefore difficult to evaluate

Table 2 (continuation)

No.	Name, Age, Sex	Basic disease	Operation (Extent of incision, length × depth)	Operat. result immed. 1	2	3	4	late 1	2	3	4	Damage of algic sensation	Complications	Notes
15	H. J. 47, w.	Causalgia manus dx.	5 × 5 mm. s. segm.	+					+			diminishing hypalges. dx. with exception of face	very mild paraesthesias slight, but frequent headache	
16a	O. B. 45, m.	Phantom pain of lower limb sin.	4 × 6 mm. dx. segm.	+ (4 days)						+		transit. hypalgesia Th 12—S 5 sin.		complete cessation of phantom pain for 48 hours, from the 5th day original intensity
16b	O. B. 45, m.	dtto.	5 × 8 mm. dx. segm.	+						+		marked hypalges. sin.	tinnitus sin., diplopia, neocerebellar symptom 14 days	return of phantom pain 4 weeks later, pain slightly less. Died two years later from apoplexy
17	M. G. 68, w.	Tabetic anorectal crises	5 × 3 mm. dx. 5 × 3 mm. s. segm.	+						+		transit. hypalges. L 3—S 5	tinnitus bilat. for 3 weeks	relief lasting only 12 days, than relapse
18	K. Sch. 59, m.	Tabetic gastric crises	4 × 6 mm. dx. 4 × 7 mm. s. segm.			+					+	marked hypalges.	severe hyperpath., tinnitus, severe impairment of hearing, diplopia	hiccup 3 days

In a majority of patients relieved from pain by the operation or with pain at least diminished, spirits rose already on the first postoperative day, patients were livelier, three of them euphoric (No. 1, 5, 14). Two patients on the contrary were sad and depressed after operation, though stating that pain had been relieved. In the first of these two patients, however, troublesome dysaesthesia appeared later. More than half the patients experienced headache after operation, as a rule of slight intensity, lasting a few days at the most. One patient (No. 15) operated for causalgia of the hand already in the year 1955 states that she suffers more frequent headaches since operation which, however, is relieved by an analgetic tablet and disappears for many hours.

Unpleasant tinnitus after operation was stated to be present in seven cases (No. 4, 6, 7, 13, 16, 17 and 18). Those who had bilateral operations (No. 6, 7, 17 and 18) also had bilateral tinnitus, with unilateral operations this was mainly on the contralateral side although sometimes also affecting the homolateral side with lesser intensity. Audiograms made after operation showed slight impairment of hearing for high tones subjectively imperceptible; however, in one case (No. 18) severe loss of hearing following bilateral segmental operation was observed (MIKULA-ŠIROKÝ-ZAPLETAL). Tinnitus persisted in these cases after unilateral interventions for a few days only and disappeared after a week at the latest; with bilateral segmental operations it persisted for 4 weeks at the most.

As regards further secondary neurological symptoms due to mesencephalic lesions, we observed in two patients (No. 16 and 18) temporary paresis of the oculomotor muscles with diplopia, returning to normal within 3 days in both cases. Five patients experienced a sensation of heaviness in the contralateral limb, however, lacking objective signs of disturbance of the pyramidal tract. One patient (No. 16) had, after operation, dysarthria and neocerebellar syndrome, characterized mainly by hypermetry. These disorders tended to recover in a fortnight. It appears that all these secondary objective signs are due to a transitory disturbance of circulation, or as the case may be, due to temporary oedema surrounding the site of destruction. Defects in cerebellar activity may be caused also by a direct partial lesion of the dentatothalamic tracts. Otherwise, these incidents described never caused serious complications of postoperative recovery and are listed only for the sake of completeness.

In some of these cases the neurologist found reduced tactile sensitivity. This was always temporary and never attained higher degrees, when the patient would be aware of this disturbance. The same applies also to deep sensitivity. Deviations from normal conditions could be found only by detailed investigations. Skin temperature values were measured in four cases, as well as oscillometric values. Both remained unaffected by the operation.

As far as the effect of mesencephalotomy on pain is concerned, this disappeared or was substantially reduced immediately after operation in 9 cases (No. 5, 7, 9 a, 12, 14, 15, 16 a, 16 b and 17), i.e. in 47.3%; in 3 cases, i.e. 15.8%, grade two improvement was recorded, in five, i.e. 26.3% operation produced no effect whatever on preoperative symptoms, in one, i.e. 5.3%, deterioration set in immediately after operation and finally one patient, i.e. 5.3% died on the fifth postoperative day. Persistent, entirely satisfactory effect on loss of pain could, however, be recorded in only 4 cases (No. 5, 7, 14 and 15), i.e. in 21%, in 3 cases (No. 1, 2 and 6), i.e. in 15.8% improvement of up to 50% was recorded, in 6 operation cases (No. 9, 10, 12, 13, 16 and 17), i.e. in 31.5% no substantial change in their condition was apparent after operation and finally in 4 cases, i.e. in 21% symptoms got worse.

In two women (No. 5 and 7) perfect relief from pain persisted up to their decease three and two and a half months respectively after operation, in the patient with the retroperitoneal teratoma (No. 14) even for 16 months. In the woman suffering from causalgia of her right hand (No. 15) relief persisted up to the date of writing, which means for 9 years after operation. There is slight hemihypalgesia of the entire half of the body excluding the face and the patient has mild tactile hyperpathia in the region of the scar following metacarpal amputation. However, this woman continues to feel much better than before operation, is employed and works even with the affected hand, whereas before the operation any touch caused her intolerable pain. As a result she was not even capable of looking after herself and became a prey to severe mental depression. The postoperative course in this woman with causalgia and sequelae of mesencephalic tractotomy after a prolonged time interval reveals the shortcomings in our knowledge on the pathophysiology of central pain. It confirms that the mechanisms responsible for the origin of these complaints are still more complicated than those for somatic pain, and also that they demand for their relief the exclusion of other afferent sections than the spinothalamic tract, as already pointed out by TALAIRACH et al.

As is shown by the table of mesencephalotomies, a majority of patients underwent only segmental incisions with additional undermining of the brachium in order to preserve as many fibres of the hearing pathway as possible. The majority of operations was performed at a higher level than is WALKER's intercollicular plane. This "superior" segmental mesencephalic tractotomy frequently achieves only hypalgesia rather than analgesia of the appropriate part of the body, however, pain may be controlled adequately at least for a time. This was also the case with patients No. 5 and 7. In the second woman a more extensive transection of the lower brachium was done, tinnitus was its result. Undermining of the brachium during this type of intervention appears fully justified. Particularly in bilateral operations, preservation of the major portion of lateral lemniscus fibres is of paramount importance, if we wish to avoid serious complications such as hearing loss and symptoms complained of by our case No. 18. As already mentioned, "lateral" segmental incisions are more easy technically, than "medial", the latter were used for eliminating pain solely in the upper part of the body. On the other hand, of course, we cannot hope to secure permanent analgesia and persisting effect with the lateral segmental incision, in view of the fact that the reticular formation with its secondary pain pathways is left entirely intact.

Hyperpathia was the most frequent complication also in our patients. It affected a total of nine patients, i. e. 47.3%, very severe in four (No. 3, 4, 8 and 18), i. e. 21% and more troublesome than the original pain. The incidence of hyperpathia in the writer's series, however, indicates that there exists no strict indirect correlation with the extent of the incision, or at least that limited destruction is not the sole factor responsible for the origin of hyperpathia. This occurred, as is revealed by the Tables, after small incision (No. 8) in accordance with contemporarily recognized functional theories of long direct and indirect pain pathways, as well as after more extensive incisions (No. 4, 18). It appears that a small "selective" segmental incision is unable to eliminate completely painful afferance from the desired region of the body, however, it may frequently be sufficient for relieving pain at least for a period of several weeks. Such a period is, as a rule sufficient as regards treatment of pain accompanying malignancies. This was finally also one of the reasons why the writer, during the next phase of operations on the stem, shifted the destruction site towards the borderline between mesencephalon and thalamus, where the pain pathways are concentrated into a narrower space.

4. Stereotactic Mesencephalotomy

Stereotactic mesencephalotomy is performed mainly by SPIEGEL and WYCIS, also by ROEDER and ORTHNER, MAZARS and finally LEKSELL. According to their descriptions these operations are performed at the level of the corpus geniculatum mediale, i.e. at the juncture of mesencephalon and thalamus which means that they are in fact mesencephalothalamotomies.

The latest paper by Wycis and Spiegel, published in 1962, reports long-term results in 54 patients who were submitted to mesencephalotomy, or a combination of this intervention with destruction of the dorsomedial nucleus. The writers, in their description of individual cases, do not always state, whether operation concerned only the mesencephalon, or whether the dorsomedial thalamic nucleus was destroyed simultaneously. The writers operated 7 cases with atypical trigeminal neuralgia. A good result was obtained in one woman who has been symptomfree for 13 years already. Out of seven patients with postherpetic pain, one has been free of symptoms for 8 years following mesencephalothalamotomy, another experienced about 50% relief for 3 years. Tabetic crises in two patients were only temporarily controlled for 9 and 8 weeks respectively. These writers also operated 6 patients for spastic pains following spinal cord injury. One was permanently relieved of pain following mesencephalotomy, a second following mesencephalothalamotomy, a third experienced only temporary relief. Out of 11 patients operated for pain due to malignant neoplasm four achieved an excellent or satisfactory result, partial improvement occured in another three. A total of 16 cases were operated for thalamic syndrome. Good and lasting results were seen in five, whereas six suffered relapse of pain after 1 to 5 months. One operation in the mesencephalon was performed for pontine haemorrhage and another for aneurysm of the a. communicans anterior, with excellent result. Only a single case of phantom pain was submitted to operation with resulting relief from pain persisting already for 10 years, in another case with causalgia, hyperpathia originated later.

Roeder and Orthner (1961) concentrated their attention during their stereotactic interventions in the midbrain on the "medial" mesencephalon. The object of their operation was the disintegration, as complete as possible, of the dorsal portion of the reticular formation of the mesencephalon. These writers perform either isolated medial destruction, or combine this step with transection of the spinothalamic bundle in the mesencephalon; this they call "lateral" mesencephalotomy. Medial operation controlled also arterial hypertension in one female patient and for a time Parkinson's syndrome. Both writers have so far performed 9 mesencephalotomies and another four they combined with destruction of the dorsomedial nucleus.

With regard to complications following stereotactic operations in the mesencephalon, Spiegel and Wycis state that they saw up to 50% incidence of audiographic changes and hearing disturbances up to the time of performing destruction at the level of the inferior colliculus. In patients in whom coagulation was done at the level of the superior colliculus the incidence of acoustic impairment dropped to 16.6%. Hyperpathias originated in only 14.8%. In five patients disturbances of motor activity occurred, permanent hemiparesis in one. Three times they registered partial paresis of the third cranial nerve, three instances of Parinaud's syndrome, two of them permanent. Extrapyramidal disturbances occurred in five cases, mental upset in two, once after mesencephalotomy, once after mesencephalothalamotomy. Immediate postoperative mortality amounted to 7.4%. These are better overall results than those achieved in the 31 cases treated by open operation and listed in the monograph by WHITE and SWEET where mortality was 16.1%. However, out of our 19 cases of open mesencephalotomies only a single patient died, a mortality of 5.3%.

WYCIS and SPIEGEL thus prefer stereotactic mesencephalotomy to open operation, stressing the lower mortality as well as the smaller percentage of complications. Most striking is the low percentage of postoperative hyperpathias, a fact which can only partly be explained by destruction at the juncture of mesencephalon and thalamus. More frequent complications from the region of the oculomotor nerves and their nuclei as well as from the extrapyramidal region, however, indicate that the lesion set by stereotaxis is after all less accurate and as a rule more extensive and may more easily affect neighbouring structures, than is the case with open intervention. The occurrence too of persisting pyramidal disturbances and mental disorders are evidence of greater and more frequent deviation from the correct site of destruction. The most dangerous sequelae are, of course, a result of erroneous destruction taken too far medially and ventrally. Lesions set partly in these areas were probably also instrumental in the origin of extrapyramidal disturbances.

5. The Open Mesencephalothalamotomy

In another series of 14 patients operated during the 1958—1960 period destruction of painful pathways was performed at the junction of mesencephalon and thalamus, where the painful spinothalamic tract, already considerably thinned, is concentrated in the smallest space. At this juncture, called porta thalami by HASSLER, the pain pathway is deflected laterally and dorsally, enlarging conically into the nucleus ventrocaudalis parvocellularis.

As already stated in the chapter on surgical technique, destructions at these levels were also done with a curved scalpel with a one-sided cutting edge, the scalpel, however, was inserted at the landmark where brachium-c.g.m. meet. Table 3 enclosed shows drawings indicating the direction and extent of destruction in each operation. Here segmental destructions were performed too. In cases of pain affecting the lower part of the body, the section of the circle described by the scalpel was laterally and ventrally from the landmark. In cases where pain affected the upper part of the body, the medioventral section was destroyed. Here, as well as in lateral destruction, already also part of the truncothalamic system was affected with reticulothalamic pathways, represented mainly by the nucleus limitans placed in a lateral position.

A total of 16 mesencephalothalamotomies was performed in these 14 patients. Lateroventral destruction was done in 10 of them, on account of pain in the lower half of the body, and medioventral in four, for pain in the upper half of the body. In three patients with rectal cancer metastases and circumanal pain (No. 22, 23 and 30), as well as in patient No. 19 with hypernephroma metastases, also upper thoracic chordotomy was done on the opposite side, in addition to mesencephalothalamotomy (MT) for bilateral pain. Both these operations were done in a single stage in a sitting position. In another patient (No. 29) chordotomy on the right was done first for metastatic pain in the left side, five weeks later also left MT. The patient, despite marked hypaesthesia, continued to demand the administration of opiates after operation, as a result of addiction. For this reason destruction of the dorsomedial nucleus on the left was done a fortnight later in addition. However, severe frontal symptomatology ensued, persisting practically unabated right up to death which took place two months later. No further pain was complained of by this patient for his remaining period of survival. Reoperation after two and 15 days respectively with more extensive destruction was done in another two cases (No. 19 and 20), on account of failure of the first incision made at the borderline between mesencephalon and thalamus.

There were 12 males and two females amongst the 14 operation cases. Of these, eleven were suffering from pain due to metastases. Six patients had cancer of the rectum, one had cancer of the pelvic colon, one a hypernephroma, one gastric cancer, one lung cancer and finally one woman had a cervical neuroblastoma. One other case, a male, had spastic pains accompanying amyotrophic lateral sclerosis, another thalamic syndrome and finally a woman aged 70 years, the oldest in this group, was suffering from postherpetic

Table 3. *Mesencephalothalamotomy*

No.	Name, Age, Sex	Basic disease	Operation (Extent in mm.)	Operat. result immed. 1	2	3	4	late 1	2	3	4	Damage of algic sensation	Complications	Notes
9b	F. K. 54, m.	Ca. recti St. p. mesencephaloto-miam dx.	9 *sin*	+				+				marked hypalges. C 2—S 5	numbness of limbs	circumanal pain decreased
10b	F. P. 46, m.	Ca. recti St. p. mesencephaloto-miam sin.	8 *sin*	+				+				marked hypalges. Th 10—S 5, mild C2—Th10	coldness and deadness of lower limb dx., reduction of vibrat. sensat.	
19a	J. R. 41, m.	Tu. Grawitzi dx.	7 *sin*			+		+				hypalges. 6 h. only	slight dysaesthes. dx., mild hemiparesis	plus chordotomy dx. died 8 weeks later
19b			9 *sin*	+								marked hypalges. dx. C 1—S 5		
20a	E. L. 64, m.	Tu. pleurae	7 *sin*			+		+				hypalges. dx. 24 h.	numbness, clumsiness, diplopia	dermolexy reduced died 7 weeks later
20b			9 *sin*	+								analgesia to Th 10, hypalgesia to S 5		

Table 3 (continuation)

No.	Name, Age, Sex	Basic disease	Operation (Extent in mm.)	Operat. result immed.				Operat. result late				Damage of algic sensation	Complications	Notes
				1	2	3	4	1	2	3	4			
21	J. F. 60, m.	Amyotrophic lateral sclerosis	7 sin		+					+		hypalges. mainly on acral parts of limbs		painful strangling pressure uncontrolled
22	J. F. 59, m.	Ca. recti	8 sin	+								mild hypalges. dx.	tracheostomy on the 8th day post oper., light psychic alter., impairment of hearing	plus chordotomy dx. died 25th day post oper. from bronchopneumonia
23	A. H. 45, m.	Ca. recti	8 sin		+				+			hypalges. dx.	slight reduction of hearing	plus chordotomy dx. died 14 weeks later
24	L. Š. 45, m.	Ca. sigmoidei	8 sin		+					+		mild hypalges. dx.		6 weeks without pain, afterwards circumanal pain, died 4 months later
25	K. B. 54, m.	Ca. recti	8 dx		+				+			analgesia to Th 12, hypalges. Th 12—S 5 sin.	mild hyperpathias	died 3 months later

Table 3 (continuation)

No.	Name, Age, Sex	Basic disease	Operation (Extent in mm.)	Operat. result immed. 1	2	3	4	late 1	2	3	4	Damage of algic sensation	Complications	Notes
26	J. F. 50, m.	Thalamic syndrome dx.	sin 8		+				+			analgesia up to Th 10, hypalges. to S5	initially slight, than gradually increasing burning in upper limb	using analgetics and neuroplegics
27	K. G. 70, w.	Postherpetic syndrome intercostal dx.	sin 9		+					+		hypalges. dx., more in upper part of the body	mild hemiparesis dx., pupil dx. slightly larger	intensity of pain less, complete disappearance of severe tactile hyperalgesia
28	A. K. 16, w.	Neuroblastoma colli l. sin.	dx 9		+							marked hypalges. sin.	dysaesthesia mainly of upper left limb	improved, no longer on opiates, died 3 weeks later from bronchopneumonia
29	A. F. 49, m.	Ca. ventric. St. p. hepatectomiam	sin 9		+ (4 days)							marked hypalges. dx.		plus chordotomy dx., plus thalamotomy n. dorsomed., afterwards psych. alter., died 2 months later
30	V. Š. 30, m.	Ca. recti	dx 8	+						+		marked hypalges. sin.	loss of all qualities of sensation	plus chordotomy sin., died 9 weeks later from cachexia

pain. The youngest patient was the second female, aged 16 years who had the cervical neuroblastoma.

None of these fourteen patients died during the postoperative phase. None of them suffered any serious peroperative or postoperative complications, case No. 22 had tracheotomy done on the second postoperative day on account of stridorous breathing, the tube could be removed on the seventh day. Amongst disturbances in the psychic sphere, case No. 19 following extensive MT developed persisting euphoria, patient No. 20 unusual contentment and good spirits, persisting right up to death after 7 weeks, in case No. 22 on the eighth postoperative day slight, transitory loss of orientation. Severe frontal symptomatology in case No. 29 developed after unilateral destruction of the dorsomedial nucleus in the thalamus. This sequel of dorsomedial thalamotomy was also confirmed by RIECHERT's observation that such, even unilateral intervention may be followed by the same syndrome as commonly seen after bilateral frontal lobotomy. In two patients of this group (No. 19 and 27) slight, but persistent contralateral hemiparesis was observed. Patient No. 20 developed transitory diplopia and patient No. 27 slight mydriasis on the opposite side. It should be noted in this connection that ocular disturbances originated always after medioventral incisions.

None of the fourteen cases who were submitted to MT developed tinnitus or other acoustic sensations, however, in two patients (No. 22 and 23) slight perceptive deafness could be diagnosed. This originated in all probability as a sequel of a lesion in the anterior and medial segments of the c.g.m. Only exceptionally could impairment of other qualities of sensitivity be observed in this group—other than algic and temperature—but these were never fully developed. In patients No. 10 b and 20 b transitory impairment of tactile discrimination and vibration was found, and in case No. 30 impairment of all qualities of sensibility, despite the fact that the incision did not belong to the most extensive interventions in this region.

As is revealed by Table 3, a satisfactory operation result with disappearance of pain was observed immediately after surgery in six cases (No. 9 a, 10 b, 19 b, 20 b, 22 and 30), i.e. 37.5%. In two of these repeated operation was necessary to achieve the result. Substantial diminution of pain and improvement of the general condition occured in 8 operation cases (No. 21, 23, 24, 25, 26, 27, 28 and 29), i.e. in 50%. In the last case improvement was of only four days duration. In two patients who failed to benefit from the first operation (No. 19 a and 20 a), reoperation MT was done after two and fifteen days respectively. A permanent result was recorded in four patients (No. 9 b, 10 b, 19 b and 20 b), i.e. in 25%; in three cases (No. 23, 25 and 28), i.e. 18.75% pain was relieved up to 50%, in another two patients (No. 22 and 27) only slight improvement compared with the preoperative state was registered, in patient No. 26 with thalamic syndrome more marked improvement was marred by dysaesthesias of the upper limbs, the condition remained unchanged after operation in three cases (No. 21, 24 and 30). Patient No. 29 was allocated to grade 3 in the Table of permanent results, however, in view of the emergence of fairly severe frontal symptomatology after destruction of the medial thalamic nucleus the overall result was deterioration.

Marked hyperpathias complicated the outcome of MT only in a single instance, case No. 26, whereas only dysaesthesias were present in cases 19 b, 21, 25 and 28, exceeding only somewhat the usual pattern of sensory changes which takes place in patients with tractotomies on the trunk.

MT, as may be seen, appears to offer some advantages as compared with simple mesencephalotomy. The most remarkable is the low percentage of postoperative hyperpathias. Perhaps a significant role in this respect is played by transection of the truncothalamic system during MT, represented here by the section of the portal part of nucleus limitans. The insignificant incidence of acoustic complications may be understood easily if we bear in mind the site of the lesion. Only at times is the anterior portion of the c.g.m. involved with resulting minor acoustic disturbances.

As revealed by the Tables, segmental interventions, either intercollicular or at the porta thalami, achieved in the majority of cases mere hypalgesia. Despite the fact, that pain was adequately controlled in many, skin algesia returned to normal so rapidly during the ensuing weeks that further effect could not be counted upon. The present writer avoided more extensive destruction in this region, capable of producing analgesia, on account of the possible emergence of acoustic disturbances as well as hyperpathias, and the danger of oculomotor, motor and vegetative disorders.

The writer, for the reasons advanced, performed destruction of the thalamic nucleus ventrocaudalis parvocellularis and the truncothalamic system nuclei in the next section, again employing an open approach. The growing number of promising results of other writers provided the stimulus. They performed destruction in the thalamus first in "central", later also in somatic intractable pain.

This last group comprises 22 patients who had antalgic operations in the thalamus done. These operations are done elsewhere in the world, with the exception of the writer, exclusively by stereotaxis.

6. Stereotactic Thalamotomy

The era of thalamic surgery for pain was inaugurated by SPIEGEL and WYCIS who exploited the findings of FREEMAN and WATTS. The latter saw, after frontal lobotomies, a change in the mental reaction to pain. WATTS noticed already in 1936 that a female patient submitted to bilateral leucotomy for severe psychoneurosis, was relieved of pain in the lumbar region which had troubled her extremely before operation. The selfsame writer was also the first to perform, in the year 1943 frontal leucotomy for pain. SPIEGEL and WYCIS (1950, 1953) decided accordingly, to perform in patients with severe pain, with the affective components in the foreground, destruction of the dorsomedial nucleus of the thalamus where thalamofrontal pathways project. The sequelae of dorsomedial thalamotomy vary and are governed mainly by the extent of destruction of the medial nucleus. Experience showed that the antalgic effect of such an operation is directly proportional to the psychological effect on the patient. This is a conclusion similar to that applying to frontal leucotomy. For these reasons destruction of the entire dorsomedial nucleus has been abandoned at present, particularly as it became clear that such a, even unilateral, operation may result in the emergence and persistence of severe frontal symptomatology. Also SPIEGEL and WYCIS perform only partial destruction of the dorsomedial nucleus, frequently in combination with destruction of the spinothalamic tract in the mesencephalon. The writer, in cases with marked affective component of pain, employs at present a new technique, consisting of partial transection of the frontothalamic pathways in the thalamus, the so-called partial longitudinal thalamotomy, as described in the previous chapter on surgical technique.

ROEDER and ORTHNER (1961) perform destruction of the nucleus centralis thalami and its surroundings in the conviction that such interventions interrupt a much greater number of spinothalamic fibres than the simple lesion of n. v. c. pc. They consider, accordingly, destruction of this nucleus as essential for the good effect of thalamotomy.

Destruction of the termination of the spinothalamic tract in the thalamus, n. v. c. pc., was first done by TALAIRACH and coworkers. These writers reported operation of 12 cases for thalamic syndrome. In six, i. e. 50%, they observed disappearance or substantial reduction of pain, in two, i. e. 16% pain was partly suppressed and the general condition was improved by about 50%, in another two cases only slight relief was registered and finally the last two cases died during the postoperative phase. The writers stress that results achieved were surprisingly good, if only on account of the advanced age of their patients ranging between 53 and 75 years. In their opinion the good effect was not purely a result of destruction of the n. v. c. pc.—in any case not always complete—in view of the fact that skin sensibility for pain was frequently only diminished. They conclude that thalamotomy will be most suitably indicated in the presence of thalamic pains and that it is not likely to be effective in peripheral pain. Nevertheless growing experience and advances in stereotactic technique led to increasingly frequent use of thalamotomy also for somatic pains, mainly those due to malignancies.

SPIEGEL, WYCIS and FREED (1952) likewise performed the so-called ventrolateral thalamotomy, however, no detailed and documented analysis is contained in their paper.

MONNIER up to the year 1955 performed with various collaborators 10 destructions of n. v. c. pc. Detailed reports of four operations done in three patients are published in his paper. In the first two who had rather "limited" coagulation the effect lasted for 2—3 months. Both patients were suffering from atypical trigeminal neuralgia. Transitory slight hemiparesis occured also in the first operation case, in the second MONNIER decided, on account of the shortlived effect, to perform more extensive thalamotomy, than at the first session, also on the opposite side. This operation resulted in loss of pain lasting five months, however, slight but persisting spastic hemiparesis as well as ageusia, thalamic syndrome and vegetative disturbances appeared. In the last case, MONNIER performed coagulation of n. v. c. pc. and n. centralis thalami for causalgia of the arm. Relief from pain lasted 10 months, hemiparesis likewise emerged as a complication in this case, mainly affecting the tips of limbs, as well as slight mental upset.

HASSLER with RIECHERT, in their paper published 1959, describe experiences with 24 operations in the thalamus done for pain. Immediate results were excellent in four-fifths of cases, however, in 50%, partial or even complete relapse occured later. The authors recorded 8.2% mortality. As regards complications: three instances of transitory paresis, one permanent paresis of the lower limb, one instance of temporary motor aphasia and one case of temporary ataxia. RIECHERT (1960) concludes from his results that the best antalgic effect of thalamotomy may be expected if this is associated with the development of skin analgesia. In such cases, however, paralysis of extremities is common. The high percentage of failures is caused on one hand by the complex nature of the painful syndrome, on the other by the anatomical conditions unfavourable for stereotaxis. This writer also stresses in his paper (1960) that

stereotactic thalamotomy should be reserved only for cases where
all other methods proved failures. Stereotaxis of Parkinsonism is,
according to RIECHERT, much more rewarding and not associated
with so many complications. Only the future will tell whether mesencephalotomy is preferable to thalamotomy.

According to a literary report, RIECHERT performed 52 operations up to the end of the year 1964 on thalamus for pain, i.e. 9
for thalamic syndrome, 10 for posttraumatic plexitis and visceral
pain, 17 for phantom and causalgic pain and 16 for anaesthesia
dolorosa. However, the late results are not known to me.

ROEDER and ORTHNER (1961) likewise observed in their patients
after thalamotomy persisting hemipareses and even the development of Parkinson's syndrome, due, in the writers opinion at least,
to a lesion of the substantia nigra.

BETTAG and YOSHIDA published the largest series of thalamotomies for pain. In their paper published in 1960, these authors
report the results of 41 operations in 36 patients, at the neurological
congress in Zürich held in 1960 they presented their results with
52 destructions of various thalamic nuclear complexes (after RÖDER
and ORTHNER, 1961).

Out of the 36 patients of BETTAG and YOSHIDA seven were operated for anaesthesia dolorosa. One patient died from thalamic haemorrhage, the immediate postoperative result was satisfactory in
the remaining six cases, however, dysaesthesias recurred after 8—12
weeks in five patients. In four of these pain was less severe and of
a somewhat altered character. Accordingly, these writers performed
in one female patient destruction of the nucleus centralis thalami
and nucleus dorsomedialis. Pain persisted, but antalgic drugs could
be reduced. Four cases were suffering from thalamic pains. The
writers destroyed the n.v.c.pc. in three, n. dorsomedialis in one.
Two were permanently cured from pain, one only temporary. Pain
persisted in the case with destruction of n. dorsomedialis, however,
the general condition improved. Another four patients had surgery
for postherpetic neuralgia. Permanent relief was obtained in two,
temporary in one, the last patient died on the tenth postoperative
day from pneumonia. Six patients had stump and phantom pains.
Excellent results were obtained in all, however, only as far as stump
pain was concerned. Phantom pain disappeared only for a short
period, it recurred after 2—3 months at the latest. A slight, but
permanent effect was achieved only in two cases, however, mental
alterations accompanied this. Amongst another 11 cases operated
for phantom pain destruction of n.v.c.pc. was done in eight, of the
n. centralis thalami in one, of the n. centralis thalami and n. dorso-

medialis in one and solely of the n. dorsomedialis also in one case. No lasting satisfactory results were obtained in seven out of the group of eight cases. Control of pain was best and most durable after destruction of the n. centralis thalami. The n. v. c. pc. was destroyed in only four cases on account of pain due to malignancy. Immediate results were excellent. One patient died after four weeks, one after six weeks, late results were unsatisfactory in the remaining two cases. BETTAG and YOSHIDA observed phatic disorders in five cases, transitory in twelve. Out of 36 operation cases two, i. e. 5.6% died after operation. These writers believe that destruction of the n. v. c. pc. will probably emerge as the optimal thalamic intervention for pain, in combination with destruction of the n. dorsomedialis. The n. centralis thalami, according to the writers, should be transected, because it represents an important component of the truncothalamic system.

MARK with ERVIN and HACKETT (1960) performed 19 antalgic thalamic operations in 17 patients. Fourteen of them were suffering from pain due to malignancy, one had dysaesthesias following injury of the cervical cord, one had phantom pains of the upper limb, one postherpetic facial pain. These writers implant electrodes in the thalamus and leave them in place for a period of several weeks, even months. Coagulation is thus possible when required and may be further extended.

It is noted with interest that in eleven cases of MARK et al. relief from pain occurred already after mere introduction of electrode into the ventrocaudal nucleus, from mere mechanical damage, as a rule lasting only a few days, in one case, however, for 5 months. In two other cases who had electrodes inserted into the dorsomedial nucleus, a painless state ensued for two and one day respectively. These writers frequently observed, even after unilateral operations, temporary depression, desorientation and apathy in one case, after a more extensive unilateral operation even unconsciousness lasting for eight days. Temporary paresis developed in three cases, persisting monoplegia in one. Three patients died 8, 17 and 2 days after operation, two from infection, one from haemorrhage from the gastrointestinal tract. Their mortality amounted to 17.6%. As a rule only hypalgesia was achieved by electrodestruction, however, substantial relief from pain was observed by them in 13 cases with malignancies. They observed protracted relief from pain in three patients with cancer pain from larynx and tongue, despite the absence of sensibility loss in these cases. In their view this subjective relief is due to destruction of other thalamic structures than those where sensory pathways terminate. Such an effect without objective disturbances of sensibility was also observed in one case with cancer of the tongue after destruction of the dorsomedial nucleus.

COOPER (1965) in his paper presents experiences with thalamotomy in 33 cases. Twenty-one of them experienced relief after operation, i.e. 64%. However, only 11 still admitted relief after six months. Mortality was nil. Eight patients had surgery for thalamic pain. In six of them immediate relief was observed by COOPER, however, this number was reduced to only two after three months. Operation was effective mainly after destruction of VPL, VPM and centrum medianum. In four patients with phantom pain relief from phantom and pains was experienced by all and this still persisted in three cases two months after operation. Two of these cases had bilateral interventions, as pains returned after unilateral operation. It is noted with interest that the phantom disappeared already after unilateral operation, pains, however, returned. This contrasts somewhat with our personal observation. We observed, as a rule, return of the phantom after thalamotomy with persisting relief from pain. The paper does not state to what degree algesia was affected by the operation. Two patients continued to suffer from atypical facial pain. In both cases a good effect was observed by the writer for a period of six months. In this instance nucleus arcuatus and centrum medianum were destroyed. Likewise, in two patients with causalgic pain a favourable effect was achieved which lasted for over one year. Surprising are the relatively unsatisfactory results of thalamotomy in metastatic pains. Only two out of twelve cases operated by the writer had satisfactory results. It is concluded, therefore, that thalamotomy in central pain offers greater expectations for success than in somatic pain. As opposed to MARK et al., COOPER failed to see any defect of sensation with freezing of nucleic centers, solely a decrease in acuity of perception of two-points discrimination. The cases experienced subjectively sensations of tingling and numbness in the corner of the mouth and fingers.

7. The Open Thalamotomy

The present writer performed a total of 30 operations on the thalamus for intractable pain in 22 patients, 7 females and 15 males (Table 4). Pain due to neoplastic conditions was concerned in 17 cases. Pain was due to metastatic breast cancer in four women, two men had malignancies of the neck, one male a neuroblastoma of the thoracic region, one man had cancer of the lungs, another four men metastases of gastric cancer, one woman uterine cancer with metastases, one man sarcoma of the shoulder, one man sarcoma of the os

Table 4. *Thalamotomy*
(r. v. c. pc., n. dorsomedialis, partial longitudinal thalamotomy)

No.	Name, Age, Sex	Basic disease	Operation	Operat. result								Damage of algic sensation	Complications	Notes
				immed.				late						
				1	2	3	4	1	2	3	4			
31	L. N. 53, w.	Ca. mammae sin.	v. c. pc. med., partial longitudin. thalamotomy dx.	+					+			marked hypalges. sin.	slight euphoria. temporary hypogeusia	lost anorexia, two months later pain in the spine and right chest, died 11 months later
32	F. M. 57, w.	Ca. mammae dx.	v. c. pc. med.	+				+				analgesia dx.	slight euphoria	without pain surviving 12 months postoperat.
33	M. Z. 43, w.	Ca. mammae sin.	v. c. pc. med. and midle part, part. longitud. thalamotomy	+				+				analgesia sin. excluding face		without pain up to death 8 weeks later
34	M. K. 51, w.	Ca. mammae dx.	v. c. pc. med.	+				+				analgesia to the symphysis	slight diffuse tingling in the elbow and shoulder dx.	without pain living 14 months after operation
35	A. P. 64, m.	Sa. colli dx.	v. c. pc. med. sin.	+						+		marked hypalges. mostly in face	tactile hypaesthesia, corneal dx. reduced, mild ataxia, hypogeusia dx.	4 weeks without pain, than opiates again died 5 months later
36	K. O. 58, m.	Blastoma colli dx.	v. c. pc. med. and midle part, partial longitudinal thalamotomy	+					+			analgesia only in the face, hypalges. else	mild euphoria, tracheostomy 10 days, mild dysaesthesia and hypogeusia dx.	died 10 weeks later

Table 4 (continuation)

No.	Name, Age, Sex	Basic disease	Operation	Operat. result immed. 1	2	3	4	late 1	2	3	4	Damage of algic sensation	Complications	Notes
37	J. G. 58, m.	Sa. extremit. super. sin.	v.c.pc. dx.	+				+				analgesia sin.	slight decrease of corneal reflex, tactile sensibil., hypogeusia	without pain surviving 11 months postoperat.
38	J. S. 19, m.	Blastoma thorac. dx.	v.c.pc. med. sin.	+				+				marked hypalges. more in upper parts	temporary ataxia	up to death 4 months later without pain
39	A. K. 47, m.	Ca. pulm.	v.c.pc. med. dx.	+								hypalges. dx.		died per operat. of air embolism
40	A. K. 54, m.	Ca. ventric.	chemothalamot. v.c.pc. sin., destruct. n. doromed. dx.	+								hypalges. dx.	mild apathy, impairment of hearing, slight on left	drug addict, died three months later
41	J. K. 52, m.	Ca. ventric.	v.c.pc. dx., partial longitudinal thalamotomy dx.	+						+		analgesia sin.	euphoria, temporary ataxia, hypodiadochokinesis sin., diplopia	died two months later
42	J. D. 52, m.	Ca. ventric.	v.c.pc. dx.	+				+				analgesia		plus chordotomy sin., died on the 10th day post operat. from bronchopneumonia
43	V. Š. 32, w.	Ca. uteri	v.c.pc. sin.	+				+				marked hypalges.	temporary apathy, headache, tracheostomy for one week	plus chordotomy dx., died 10 weeks later
44	J. M. 53, m.	Sa. ossis pubis	chemothalamotomy v.c. sin.											died on the 2nd day post operat. from vegetative disturbances

Table 4 (continuation)

No.	Name, Age, Sex	Basic disease	Operation	Operat. result immed.				Operat. result late				Damage of algic sensation	Complications	Notes
				1	2	3	4	1	2	3	4			
45	A. S. 43, m.	Ca. recti	v. c. pc. lat. dx.	+					+			analgesia	numbness in the lower left extremity	plus chordotomy sin., using analgetics
46	R. S. 26, w.	Ca. recti	v. c. pc. dx.	+				+				analgesia	severe headache 3 days	plus chordotomy sin., living, much improved
47	F. P. 68, m.	Thalamic syndrome sin.	v. c. pc. dx., partial longitudinal thalamotomy dx.	+						+		marked, later diminishing hypalges. to Th 12	desorientation 12 hours post operat.	subj. complaints relieved only slightly
48	M. S. 60, w.	Anaesthesia dolorosa dx.	v. c. pc. sin. partial longitudinal thalamotomy sin.	+						+		diminishing hypalges. dx.	mild miosis dx. bilateral, Parinaud's syndrome, temporary ataxia	only slight subj. improvement
49	R. A. 40, m.	Phantom limb (upper extr. sin.)	v. c. pc. med. and midle part	+						+		analgesia to the umbilicus		temporarily improved, severe thalamic syndrome after stereotactic thalamotomy
50	J. K. 63, m.	Phantom limb (upper extr. dx.)	v. c. pc. sin. partial longitudinal thalamotomy sin.	+					+			analgesia to Th 11, hypalges. to S 5	slight reduction of tactile sensibil.	without pain, numbness in the right lower extremity
51	L. Š. 53, m.	Causalgia (upper right extrem.)	v. c. pc. med. sin.	+				+				analgesia to Th 10	slight dysaesthesias in the right shoulder	16 months after operation, greatly improved

pubis and two men had cancer of the rectum. Pains in another five
patients did not originate from neoplasms. One man had thalamic
syndrome, one woman suffered from anaesthesia dolorosa following
retrogasserian rhizotomy, two males had phantom and one causalgic
pains. The youngest patient was a male aged 19 years with neuroblastoma of the chest, the oldest was a man aged 68 years with
thalamic syndrome. Of the 22 patients three, i.e. 13.6% died: the
first patient died, as already mentioned in the chapter on surgical
technique, during operation from cardiac air embolism. During
transection of the dura a small opening was created in the transverse
sinus which was not filled with blood in this place. This was immediately closed with two sutures. The condition of the patient
continued to be satisfactory so that thalamotomy was performed
without incident, and with excellent subjective and objective immediate effect. When the dural flap was turned down and stretched
by the suture prior to closure of the dura, the gap in the sinus
reopened and some air was aspirated. Collapse was rapid, followed
by coma and death. The second patient with metastases of gastric
cancer and excruciating bilateral pain died on the tenth day following thalamotomy and chordotomy from severe pneumonia. His
pains were relieved up to the moment of death. The third patient
was a male aged 53 years with sarcoma metastases of the os pubis.
He died on the second postoperative day. This was the very first
patient submitted to operation in the thalamus. Chemothalamotomy had been done in this case. A fine polyethylene catheter with
inflatable balloon was inserted into the n.v.c. and 0.4 ml procain
instilled. Already following instillation of procain, the patient commenced to sweat and became strikingly apathetic. Vegetative disorders grew gradually worse after operation, coma ensued and the
patient died 46 hours after operation. Necropsy revealed general
oedema of the brain, procain destruction of the entire ventrocaudal
nucleus, of the centrum medianum and part of the dorsomedial nucleus. It is not certain, whether these serious disorders were caused
solely by extensive destruction of the posterior thalamus. We
know, that the nucleus centralis thalami belongs with its surroundings likewise to the "activating" systems (MORUZZI and MAGOUN,
1949) and influences consciousness and other vital functions. Perhaps, apart from the action of procain, an important role was also
played by an impairment of vascular supply. COOPER in the course
of his chemopallidotomies or chemothalamotomies instilled a somewhat smaller amount of procain or alcohol repeatedly, without
complications. The course of chemothalamotomy in our second patient was likewise uneventful. Chemothalamotomy was afterwards

abandoned and substituted by mechanical destruction with the loop scalpel.

Immediate results in all operation cases were excellent, pain disappeared completely in all. This very good effect, persisted in 9 cases (No. 32, 33, 34, 37, 38, 41, 43, 50 and 51). One woman with breast cancer metastases continued to survive twelve months (No. 32), a second woman (No. 34) 14 months, with complete relief of pain. This very good effect was observed also in a man with causalgia in the upper extremity (No. 51) and in a man with sarcoma of the shoulder (No. 37). The first patient is now 16 months, the second 11 months after thalamotomy. The patient No. 50 is now three and a half years after thalamotomy relieved of pain and has only very slight difficulties with his gait, caused by a feeling of numbness in the lower extremity. The remaining patients ridded of pain survived 8 weeks (No. 33), 4 months (No. 38), two months (No. 41) and two and a half months (No. 43) after operation. Another three patients (No. 31, 36 and 45) experienced only temporary complete relief from pain lasting two months, 10 days and 7 days respectively. The first patient died 11 months after operation. She was chiefly complaining of pain in the spine and right chest. The second case developed dysaesthesias of the right arm on the eleventh postoperative day, centred mainly around the elbow, requiring medication with analgetics and occasionally with neuroplegics. This patient died after two months from general cachexia. In the third patient numbness and a sensation of stiffness ensued, he received analgetics for this condition. His condition remaind unchanged five months after operation. Patient No. 35 with sarcoma of the neck had a recurrence of pain after a completely painless interval of four weeks, pains were of different, pricking character. About four months before death opiates had to be administered again. This patient died six months after operation. Patient No. 40 had chemodestruction of the n. v. c. pc. on the left. This patient was suffering from metastatic gastric cancer. He was free from pain two days after operation, later, however, diffuse abdominal pains on the left developed, and the destruction of the dorsomedial nucleus on the right was performed twelve days after the first operation. The patient did not complain of pain following this intervention and the painless state lasted six weeks. Afterwards symptoms recurred, affecting chiefly the left side of the abdomen and requiring increasing amounts of opiates for control. He died three months after operation. The patient with thalamic syndrome (No. 47) who had destruction of the n. v. c. pc. and partial longitudinal thalamotomy enjoyed a completely painless state for five days only. On the sixth day he again experienced throbbing of the upper limb, however, symptoms were much more tolerable than before operation and analgetics afforded satisfactory relief. This patient also suffered from advanced arteriosclerosis of the cerebral vessels, and continues to complain of various troubles demanding neuroplegics for their relief, despite the fact that he sleeps extremely well and looks perfectly healthy. In view of the hyperpathias complained of, however, he was allocated to grade 3 of the classification. Neither the patient with anaesthesia dolorosa (No. 48) experienced permanent relief. After one month the sensation of throbbing and numbness recurred in the entire half of the head and face associated with a bitter taste in the mouth and a sensation of swelling. However, this patient likewise enjoys excellent sleep without taking sedatives or hypnotics.

In cases No. 34, 37, 49, 50 and 51 thalamotomy was performed already with one type of the sliding loop scalpel with a radius of 6.5 mm. (Fig. 23) by the technique described for medial, or lateral thalamic destruction. Standard procedure for destruction was used, some cases, accordingly, having their operation at only one sitting under general anaesthesia. Detailed past histories and progress reports in these cases will be presented here. Case No. 49 has been dealth with in detail already on p. 57 and 58.

J. K., 63 years old man (No. 50) suffered a mine accident six years previously. The right upper limb was torn off his body. Phantom pain appeared after two months, gradually increasing in intensity. Treatment consisted of repeated revision of the amputation stump, without satisfactory result. For this reason destruction of n.v.c.pc. was done with its surrounding and was combined with partial longitudinal thalamotomy. Apart from perfect analgesia of the upper half of the body with marked lasting hypalgesia of the lower half, this patient exhibited also slight reduction of tactile sensibility. Two-point discrimination was symmetrical, deep sensation was not perceptibly involved. After a fortnightly period completely free from pain, the patient again complained of phantom sensation, however, considerably less painful and troublesome than before. No opiates were necessary since operation and analgetics only exceptionally. This subjective state of affairs, as well as objective evidence of complete analgesia of the whole upper half of the body persists still after three and a half years. After all this time the patient complains only of an uncertain gait caused by a sensation of numbness and alienation of the right lower extremity.

J. G., aged 58 years (No. 37) had his left arm amputated below the elbow for sarcoma three years ago. Intolerable pains developed three months ago in his left shoulder refractory to all types of conservative therapy. Thalamotomy n.v.c. with its surrounding was also performed in this case as a two-stage procedure, with stimulation of v.c. nucleus. The patient volunteered the information whilst still on the operating table that his pain had completely disappeared immediately after destruction. Analgesia of the entire half of the body resulted from the intervention with slight decrease of corneal reflex, tactile sensibility in the region of the face and shoulder, slight involvement of two-point discrimination, temporary impairment of vibration sense and hypogeusia. None of these postoperative defects, however, proved troublesome to the patient. Complete analgesia persists in this case for 11 months at the time of writing, and the patient is satisfied, despite the fact that the sarcomatous growth is now spreading to the scapular region and invading the entire shoulder girdle. Progress observed in this case appears to indicate that the best alleviation of peripheral pain with some permanency may be expected, after all, in cases with clinical appearance of analgesia of half the body. Despite perfect analgesia no troublesome sensations in the lower limb are complained of by the patient. Only direct questioning whether the limb does not appear numb and as if "alien" elicits a positive answer.

M. K., 51 years, female (No. 34) sustained an operation for breast cancer two years ago. Amputation was performed and an interval of two years without symptoms ensued. Afterwards, however, pain of rapidly increasing intensity developed in the right arm with considerable swelling. The patient got used to high doses of opiates with lessening effect. Thalamotomy v. c. and surroundings was done by single stage under general anaesthesia. Analgesia extending to the symphysis resulted with marked hypalgesia of the lower limb. The patient experiences the sensation of slight diffuse tingling in the elbow and shoulder of the affected upper limb and a feeling as if her hand "did not belong to her." However, she is no longer taking any analgetics and this good effect persists 14 months after operation.

L. Š., born 1912 (No. 51), met with an accident at the age of 11 years; amputation of the right forearm had to be done. He was symptom-free afterwards. Five months before admission spontaneous pains commenced, located first at the amputation site, later radiating to the right shoulder, increasing in intensity, of "causalgic pain type." This patient was treated with analgetics, vitamin B_{12}, neuroplegics, entirely without effect, relief during the last weeks was provided only by opiates. The patient's general condition was deteriorating and he was rapidly losing weight. In view of these facts surgical treatment for pain was recommended. Two-stage thalamotomy operation was performed. Electrostimulation of the n.v.c.pc. produced pain in the eyes, head and shoulder on the right side. The patient felt a lightning pain in the right half of his body already during insertion of the cannula. Control of sensibility during this phase revealed hypaesthesia in the right shoulder, thigh and face (confirming the findings of MARK and ERVIN). After destruction of the n.v.c. and surroundings, analgesia was found to be present in the right arm, chest, and back, considerable hypaesthesia of the face and slighter, but distinct hypalgesia of the abdominal region and lower limb. After 16 months there is numbness of the entire right half of the body, with very slight, not troublesome dysaesthesias in the right shoulder. The good subjective effect of the operation still persists, the skin analgesia described is maintained.

Two patients (No. 36 and 43) had to have tracheostomy ten and seven days respectively after operation on account of difficult and inadequate expectoration, as a preventive measure against pulmonary complications. Both patients, however, ran an otherwise entirely uneventful postoperative course and their general condition remained satisfactory throughout. Those patients who in addition had partial longitudinal thalamotomy, showed slight mental alteration bordering on euphoria. However, no other personality changes were observed and the deviation mentioned from the normal mental state was always welcome on account of the good spirits of the patient, as well as for the lack of interest in his troubles and other problems in his life. A similar condition developed also in a female patient (No. 32) who had only destruction of the n. v. c. pc. In this case operation in all likelihood also involved centrum medianum fibres and also a minute portion of frontothalamic and thalamo-frontal fibres. Similar sequelae are in any case published by almost all writers. Slight apathy and lack of self-interest occured in case No. 40 who had destruction of the n. dorsomedialis on the right at the second session. This patient complained only of impairment of hearing and the audiogram confirmed the presence of bilateral perception hypacusis, more pronounced on the right. These complaints originated probably as a result of chemothalamotomy on the left, where more diffuse penetration of the alcohol involved the acoustic pathway and the c. g. m. region. As regards disorders of oculomotor muscles and vision respectively, patient No. 41 had occasional diplopia. The extent of destruction was relatively large in this case and part of the tegmentum was probably involved in it. Partial longitudinal thalamotomy in this case was done to a depth of 19 mm. and a loop of larger radius was used for setting the lesion in the n. v. c. pc. Apart from diplopia and the euphoria already mentioned, slight impairment of mnestic function and ability to concentrate also developed. Complete hemianalgesia persisted up to death. In the patient No. 48 with anaesthesia dolorosa slight miosis on the right and bilateral lag in looking upward followed operation on the left, as well as transitory horizontal nystagmus, very marked on the first day, but rapidly diminishing. Only slight unsteadiness of the eyeballs could be observed after a fortnight. It resulted probably from involvement of the nucleus ventralis intermedius, when the loop was inserted too far forward.

Disturbances of taxis were observed more often, most marked in four cases (No. 35, 38, 41 and 48). These complications likewise were only transitory, did not reduce the wellbeing of patients affected and rapidly returned to normal after operation. Contralateral limb hypotonus, if present, was always very slight and short-lived. Hypodiadochokinesis of the upper extremity also developed in patient No. 41. Permanent defects and more marked involvement of the brachium conjunctivum were not registered. Disorders emanating from the internal capsule were not observed following open thalamotomy. Destruction of the lateral portion of v. c. pc. was associated several times with transitory hyperreflexia, motoricity, however, was never affected.

It was noted with interest how little thalamotomy affects other modes of sensibility, besides painful and temperature. Impairment of tactile sensibility does not appear as a rule. If found after opera-

Table 5. *Late results of mesencephalotomy and mesencephalothalamotomy of some authors in various kinds of pain*

Author	Number of cases	Disappear-ance	Improve-ment	Without change	Impair-ment	Death
I. Pain from malignant invasion:						
SPIEGEL and WYCIS	12	4	2	4		2
WHITE and SWEET	5	1	1	1		2
DRAKE and McKENZIE	4			2	2	
WALKER	3		2	1		
LEKSELL	2		2			
GRANT	1	1				
ZAPLETAL	23	6	6	4	5	2
II. Spasticity and radicular pain:						
SPIEGEL and WYCIS	9	2 (1-destr. of dorso-medial n.)	1 (destr. of dorso-medial n.)	6		
ZAPLETAL	1			1		
III. Tabetic crises:						
SPIEGEL and WYCIS	2			2		
ZAPLETAL	2			1	1	
IV. Anaesthesia dolorosa (D), Atypical facial neuralgia (AN), and Tic douloureux (T):						
ROEDER and ORTHNER	1 (D)		1			
SPIEGEL and WYCIS	7 (AN)	1	2	4		
MAZARS et al.	27 (T)	25 (?)		1		1
V. Postherpetic pain:						
SPIEGEL and WYCIS	7	1	2	4		
SJÖQVIST	2					2
DAVID et al.	1					1
GUIOT and FORJAZ	1					1
DRAKE and McKENZIE	1			1		
ZAPLETAL	1			1		
VI. Thalamic syndrome:						
SPIEGEL and WYCIS	16	5		9		2
WALKER	2		1			1
ROEDER and ORTHNER	1	1				
ZAPLETAL	1			1		
VII. Phantom pain and causalgia (C):						
SPIEGEL and WYCIS	2	1	1			
WALKER	1		1			
DRAKE and McKENZIE	1				1	
ZAPLETAL	2		1 (C)	1		

Table 6. *Late results of thalamotomy of some authors in various kinds of pain*

Author	Number of cases	Disappearance	Improvement	Without change	Impairment	Death
I. Pain from malignant invasion:						
MARK et al.	14	3	3	5		2
BETTAG and YOSHIDA	4	2		2		
RIECHERT	1	1				
COOPER	12	2				
ZAPLETAL	17	8	4	2		3
II. Spasticity and radicular pain:						
MARK et al.	1			1		
III. Tabetic crises:						
RIECHERT	1					1 (pulmon. embolism)
IV. Anaesthesia dolorosa (D), Atypical facial neuralgia (AN), and Tic douloureux (T):						
RIECHERT	8 (T)		6	2		
OBRADOR and BRAVO	3 (AN)		2	1		
MONNIER	2 (AN)		1		1	
COOPER	2 (AN)	2				
ZAPLETAL	1 (D)			1		
V. Postherpetic pain:						
BETTAG and YOSHIDA	4	2	1			1
MARK et al.	1		1			
VI. Thalamic syndrome:						
BETTAG and YOSHIDA	4	2		2		
RIECHERT	1		1			
HANKINSON et al.	1	1				
COOPER	8	2		6		
ZAPLETAL	1			1		
VII. Phantom pain and causalgia (C):						
BETTAG and YOSHIDA	17	1 (destruct. centrum medianum)	4	12		
RIECHERT	4	1	1	1		1
MONNIER	1 (C)		1			
MARK et al.	1			1		
COOPER	4 +2 (C)	3 2 (C)	1			
ZAPLETAL	3 (1 C)	1 (C)		2		

tion, it is partial as a rule and quickly adjusted (No. 35). Similarly graphaesthesia, tactile discrimination and vibration are affected very little and for short periods. This almost surprisingly small defect in proprioceptive sensibility can be explained, bearing in mind the site and extent of destruction, rather by the bilateral course of this pathway, than solely by the fact that fibres of the medial lemniscus terminate in the VP and its entire extent.

Hemihypogeusia could be observed in several of the patients with destruction of the nucleus arcuatus. These observations also confirm the physiological findings of PATTON et al. (1944) and of BLOM-QUIST et al. (1962) that thalamic representation of the pathway for taste is situated only in the posterior portion of the ventromedial complex, according to BLOMQUIST also bilaterally.

Marked hyperpathia did not occur in a single instance following thalamotomy. Mild dysaesthesias originated in only four cases (No. 36, 41, 45 and 50), in the first patient affecting only the upper limb, in the fourth the whole half of the body. This patient, an intelligent male, states that these sensations are in no way troublesome, but that he experiences during movement, walking or any other action uncertainty in the whole half of the body which leads to restlessness and anxiety. None of the 22 cases operated suffered from major disturbances of other types of sensibility. Slight tactile hypaesthesia resulted in patient No. 35 from destruction of the n.v.c. Symptoms of thalamic character were not observed in a single case in our series. Thalamic pain in patient No. 49 resulted from stereotactic intervention done elswhere.

The tables appended (Tables 5 and 6) list the number of operations and permanent results of those writers, who in their papers on mesencephalotomy, mesencephalothalamotomy and thalamotomy present detailed descriptions of the effect achieved by operation.

VI. Evaluation of Mesencephalotomy and Thalamotomy and Their Comparison with Other Surgical Methods

Many circumstances participate in the decision which method and which surgical technique is to-day selected by the neurosurgeon for controlling intractable pain from the upper half of the body and for central pain. His experience with some of the operations available and his predilections are decisive, as is the technical equipment and scope of his centre. It should surprise nobody that with these operations which we have in mind and which bear on such delicate structures as the spinomedullary junction, or the brain stem, much depends on the skill of the neurosurgeon, regarding the smooth course and good result; whereas one centre gets acquainted and elaborates, in due course, a certain type of operation, becoming fond of it and propagating its use as a rewarding operation, other centres may express fundamental objections and reservations against the selfsame method, or completely refuse its use. The diversity of view on the various operations as well as on approach routes and surgical tactics may be easily understood from the foregoing.

1. Operations in the Region of the Frontal Lobes

Some workers hold the view that interventions on the medulla and brain stem are always excessively grave. They draw attention to the fact that such operations are indicated chiefly in persons suffering from malignant disease with a short survival period in all probability and also in central pains, where interventions in the region of the secondary painful pathway remain problematical. They devote their attention, accordingly to less exacting operations, mainly in the region of the frontal lobes.

Bilateral frontal lobotomy for pain of a refractory nature has, of course, been definitely abandoned as a mutilating operation producing gross psychic changes. Much less extensive operations have been advocated, interrupting afferent fibres to the visceral or limbic cortical system. For instance WHITE and SWEET advocated in 1947 the interruption of only the lower quadrant of the frontal lobes, WATTS and MURPHY in 1949 limited transorbital leucotomy, LE BEAU in 1949 bilateral excision of the gyrus cinguli, SCARFF in

1950 unilateral frontal lobotomy, GRANTHAM in 1951 limited bi-medial frontal transection of the cortex etc. However, in the writer's opinion, despite these proposals of modified interventions for pain in the region of the frontal lobes made recently, such as frontal cingulumotomy after FOLTZ and WHITE (1962), or WHITE's bilateral electrocoagulation of white matter limited to small frontal sections (1962), the view of CONSTANS (1962) still holds good, namely that there is a direct correlation between the extent of lesions in the frontal lobes, relief from pain and personality disorders. Pain returns after operation pari passu with adjustment of psychic changes. In view of the small risk attached to it this operation is, in the writer's opinion, indicated solely in patients suffering from far advanced malignancies who are unsuitable for any other surgery, and in whom pain and troubles are associated with a marked emotional compo-nent.

2. The Upper Cervical Chordotomy

The operation that may be performed in the presence of upper pain at the lowest portion of the spinothalamic tract is upper cervical chordotomy. This is performed at the level of C_1 to C_3 with the object of achieving, by transection of the anterolateral bundle, analgesia of at least the distal cervical segments. This operation appears most simple at first glance, because it is not yet done on a manifold and composite structure, such as the medulla or the brain stem. Though in substance this is similar to thoracic chordotomy, however, soft as well as bony structures of the back of the neck, and also the topography of cervical roots (KAHN and RAND, 1950), nerve paths (HESSLER, 1960) and vessels (FRENCH, HAINES and OGLE, 1956), create much less favourable conditions than those pertaining to the lower spinal column and cord segments. It appears that the main reason for which upper cervical chordotomy has never achieved wider application lies in the first place in the fear of pro-ducing disorders of respiration. This would be particularly serious and dangerous especially in primary or complicating pulmonary diseases.

BELMUSTO (1963) found with his co-workers by means of the pneumotachograph that every, even unilateral, cervical chordotomy affects respiratory function. For this reason bilateral operation, even if done at different levels directly threatens life. Secondly, results achieved so far reveal that impairment of algic sensibility obtained immediately after operation, even though adequately high, only rarely persists (HORRAX and PRICE, 1954; GRANT and WOOD, 1956),

7*

as a result recurrence of pain is early and frequent (BOHM, 1960, in 50%). Finally also mortality, even after unilateral operation is relatively high (OGLE et al., 13.5%).

Transection of the anterolateral bundle at the highest spinal cord levels may be indicated and offer a chance of permanent success mainly in unilateral pain in the region of the thorax. If it is done with the object of eliminating pain also from the upper limb and neck, any incision made must be more extensive and deeper, thereby incurring the risk of serious complications. Bilateral operation done at one sitting, though in different segments, must be rejected. RIECHERT (1960) advocates its performance in two stages, one side at the C_1—C_2 level, on the other at the C_3—C_4 level.

3. Medullary Tractotomy

Another operation interrupting the secondary pain pathway in its upper levels was put forward in 1941 (SCHWARTZ and O'LEARY, 1941; WHITE, 1941). This is the so-called medullary tractotomy consisting of destruction of the pain pathway below the inferior olive, likewise in the immediate neighbourhood of the respiratory centres. The incision carried to a depth of 4 mm. causes temporary analgesia, or marked hypalgesia also of all cervical segments. Such an operation, whether performed with a scalpel (CRAWFORD), or electroprobe (SWEET et al.) always by the open method, is not as a rule followed by any striking neurological defects, with the exception of slight disorders of taxis due to damage to the ventral spinocerebellar tract. Some writers have become partial to it for these reasons (CRAWFORD, SWEET) and continue to elaborate it further.

However, impairment of algic sensibility as a rule quickly adjusts itself after an incision only 4 mm. in depth, with the result that pain recurs very soon. If we, therefore wish to achieve permanent relief from organic pains, or control central pain, it becomes necessary to deepen the incision further medially into the reticular nuclei and pathways of the medulla. Such an intervention, however, threatens the respiratory centres still more than upper cervical chordotomy. Equally serious are the possible sequelae of lesions affecting the nucleus ambiguus, followed by vocal cord paralysis, an insensitive pharynx and depression of the cough reflex, as well as severe disturbances of taxis due to a lesion of the corpus restiforme. This is revealed by CRAWFORD's papers (1947, 1953, 1960), who possesses the greatest experience with this operation and out of whose 23 patients six patients died immediately after operation, i.e. 26%, as well as by the overall figures of BIRKENFELD and FISHER (1963), according to which out of 59 so far published medullary tractotomies 10 patients died after operation, i.e. 17%. Bilateral one-stage procedures are in this region still more dangerous than upper cervical chordotomy. The patient of ADAMS and MUNRO survived bilateral operation, however, CRAWFORD's two patients died.

Medullary tractotomy, accordingly, should always be done by a surgeon of perfect training and solely under local anaesthesia under constant surveilance of the patient. It should be recommended chiefly in persons suffering from unilateral malignant pain, inclusive of the upper limb and neck. An incision to a depth of 6 mm. or more whose object is to involve also the reticular substance with its secondary painful pathways is already considerably hazardous.

4. Mesencephalic Tractotomy

In contrast to the two operations just briefly dealt with, i.e. upper cervical chordotomy and medullary tractotomy, mesencephalic tractotomy possesses the advantage that unilateral intervention in the midbrain does not affect vitally important functions. Even in cases where the incision involves unintentionally also the paramedial section of the reticular formation with part of the periaqueductal grey matter, though temporary depression of consciousness, mental alterations and paresis of oculomotor muscles develops, however, respiratory activity and other important autonomic functions remain intact. It is likewise unnecessary to harbour anxiety about the immediate sequelae of bilateral mesencephalotomy. There exist, however, other serious reasons, why this operation is not popular and commonly used. WHITE and SWEET in their monograph published in 1955 write about them verbatim:

"It is therefore our conclusion that spinothalamic tractotomy in the mesencephalon must still be regarded as an experimental procedure. While analgesia or a sufficient degree of hypalgesia can be obtained in a high proportion of cases, the risk of mortality from local oedema of the mesencephalon or temporal lobe and the danger of disagreeable residual paraesthesia are at present too great to justify the operation. Its potential value in the intractable atypical neuralgias of the face and in carcinoma of the pharyngeal region, where the vagus is an important conductor of pain, is so great that continued efforts must be made to overcome these objections. Care in preserving venous drainage from the temporal lobe and the use of radiation to produce the lesions, if they can be accurately made, may reduce postoperative hemianopsia, stupor and bleeding in the brain stem. Possibly these difficulties may be overcome by refinements in making the lesions with improved stereotactic instruments, but we see no solution to prevent the production of paraesthesia, which may be even more troublesome than the original pain."

This was due in the first place to the very difficult approach to the region of the mesencephalon for open operation which forced both writers to express such an unfavourable assessment of mesencephalic tractotomy. The high percentage of operative and postoperative complications, some of which even terminated fatally, were in reality due to the exacting occipital approach. The present writer's infratentorial route is, in this respect, already less severe, visualization improved, more physiological and also less time-consuming. Even in comparison with the approach used for upper cervical chordotomy or medullary tractotomy, the infratentorial approach for mesencephalic tractotomy appears simpler, as only hemicraniectomy of the posterior fossa is done, whilst for the aforementioned operations functionally decidedly more important bony structures must be sacrificed. During hemicraniectomy of the posterior fossa the most time-consuming phase is the chiselling away of bone from the external occipital protuberance. With stereotactic procedures, of course, similar problems due to the severity of making the approach to the midbrain are completely absent.

The second reason why WALKER's mesencephalic tractotomy after its first realization in 1942 failed to gain popularity with neurosurgeons lies in the involvement of the secondary acoustic pathways. In unilateral operations done in the classical WALKER style, the entire lemniscus lateralis with the acoustic pathway is deliberately transected. This results in temporary tinnitus affecting either one or both ears and to impairment of hearing for high tones, sometimes only detectable by audiography. Bilateral intercollicular incision results in deafness for all practical purposes. The incidence of this complication may be reduced either by making a shorter incision more superficially, in order to preserve at least a portion of the inferior brachium fibres, i.e. something related to "undermining", or a fine coagulation probe may be employed. Again, with such operations the extent of lesions set may not always be adequate and the antalgic effect only temporary. These disturbances of hearing were also the main reason for which the incision made in open operations (GUIOT and FORJAZ, ZAPLETAL) as well as in stereotaxis (SPIEGEL, LEKSELL) was shifted upwards, frequently up to the borderline between mesencephalon and thalamus. Almost complete avoidance of the acoustic pathway is, as a rule, possible in this situation. If, however, impairment of hearing develops after such operations, this is invariably slight and transitory. Its cause is most frequently some inaccuracy of destruction, also involving the terminal section of the inferior brachium and possibly part of the corpus geniculatum mediale.

The largest contribution to the negative attitude assumed towards mesencephalotomy, however, was made by the experience that hyperpathias develop frequently after interventions in this region. Whereas these complications are a rare exception in spinal chordotomies (WHITE and SWEET 4.3%), their incidence being somewhat higher after medullary tractotomy (CRAWFORD 8.5%), they are, however, very common after mesencephalotomy (WALKER 10%, DRAKE and McKENZIE 50%, the writer 47.3%). The intensity of the hyperpathias varies. Experience has shown that they may arise not only after limited destructions, but also in cases with complete and permanent analgesia. However, in the latter case it may prove difficult with some patients to distinguish between a more pronounced grade of sensation changes in the part of the body with injured afferentation and dysaesthesias proper. It must be admitted, however, in any case, that the likelihood of troublesome or even severe hyperpathias originating after intercollicular mesencephalic tractotomy is considerable.

5. Mesencephalothalamotomy

The main object of the writer's in shifting the point of destruction of the pain pathway right up to the junction of mesencephalon and thalamus was the endeavour to remove the danger of interfering with hearing, and also the desire to test, whether destruction of the pathway immediately before its termination in the thalamic nuclei will or will not be followed by a smaller incidence of hyperpathias. It seems probable that at this level also the secondary pain pathways are crowded into a smaller space, as here even limited incisions produce better results, than intercollicular mesencephalotomy. Neither are complications due to paresis of oculomotor muscles so frequent with open operations as they are with stereotaxis. By means of the latter, SPIEGEL and WYCIS perform lesions at about the identical level, the instrument for destruction, however, also traumatizing the larger area of the pretectal region. In the writer's personal series, hyperpathia after mesencephalothalamotomy occurred in a single case out of 14 patients. SPIEGEL and WYCIS likewise observed after their stereotactic "superior" mesencephalotomies the emergence of hyperpathias in not quite 15%.

Mesencephalic tractotomy in its classical intercollicular form has accordingly been abandoned already. As far as operations continue to be made in this structure, destructions are located at a higher level, most frequently at the mesencephalothalamic junction. Contemporarily, these operations are more frequently done by stereo-

taxis than by the open route. However, if we bear in mind the topography and extent of these sections of the brain stem, then we must
admit the difficulty of reaching by probe all the desired structures
of the porta thalami. In a majority of cases destruction has to be
done in several places and lesions thus set may often be unnecessar-
ily extensive and giving rise to complications, as borne out by some
papers. The writer is accordingly of the opinion that the open
approach facilitates much better control of the extent of destruction
and thereby affords fewer complications.

On the whole, however, even after the introduction of the various
modifications mentioned, operations on the midbrain have so far
not been widely applied. One of the main reasons for this are, to be
sure, the more hopeful results achieved in connection with severe
pain by stereotactic thalamotomy.

6. Stereotactic Thalamotomy

Stereotactic thalamotomy during the initial stage was reserved
for the classical central pain, i.e. the thalamic syndrome, mainly
as a result of the work of TALAIRACH et al. However, passage of time
and increasing experiences revealed that destruction of those thalamic nuclei where pain fibres terminate occupies a useful place in the
therapy of peripheral organic pain as well as offering hope of partial
success in relieving central pain. The segmental distribution of
fibres of the spinothalamic tract in the relatively wide ventrocaudal
nucleus facilitates in addition the first realistic thought of performing isolated destruction. However, further experiences are required
for devising a more accurate technique in detail.

The majority of truncothalamic system nuclei with the terminations of a considerable proportion of secondary pain pathway fibres
are located medially from the ventrocaudal nucleus, and are thus
easily accessible either stereotactically or by the open approach
devised by the writer. Nucleus limitans as well as nucleus centralis
thalami, part of the nucleus parafascicularis and, as shown on photographs of a brain preparation with thalamic lesions set by the loop
scalpel (Figs. 27, 28), the medial part of the zona incerta of the
subthalamus may be destroyed from the infratentorial approach.
In the subthalamic region also part of the indirect pain fibres terminate or pass through (HASSLER).

However, despite such destruction, a certain percentage of pain
conducting fibres remains intact. They are fibres terminating in
further nuclei of the medial involucrum, further thalamic nuclei,
such as nucleus reticularis, in the hypothalamus, globus pallidus

etc., and also fibres which during their ascending course cross to the opposite site in the medulla, pons, midbrain or even posterior commissure. Destruction of pain fibres in the nucleus reticularis, hypothalamus, etc. can not be entertained at present for understandable reasons. However, perhaps these pathways in particular are capable of producing relapses, perhaps due to them control of central and visceral pain is so difficult, and they might cause or enhance hyperpathias following thalamotomy. Experience obtained so far, however, luckily point to the fact that this last possibility i.e. the development of the thalamic syndrome after thalamotomy occurs only very sporadically and, it should be noted with interest, mainly in cases of excessively extensive or inconsiderate operations.

7. The Problem of Bilateral Interventions

In this connection it appears reasonable to mention a serious problem represented by the therapy of intractable pain located in the midline and of visceral or bilateral pain. According to experience, bilateral operation in such pains, performed at identical spinal cord levels, or in the brain stem in one stage, is always connected with an increased risk. In the case of upper thoracic or lower cervical chordotomy, the development of complications may be influenced by performing the operation at varied cord levels, between two segments. Such a bilateral operation is contemporarily done most frequently in the presence of pain in the lower half of the body. Its disadvantage is the frequent origin of troubles of micturition and defecation as well as paresis of the extremities. These occur chiefly with pain in the sacral region, where it becomes necessary to destroy also the laterodorsal portion of the cord right up the denticulate ligament, or even 1—2 mm. dorsally from it. Bilateral upper cervical chordotomy carries the risk of producing marked arterial hypotension, mainly, however, of oedema affecting the respiratory centres. Still greater is this same danger in bilateral medullary tractotomy. Bilateral operations in the mesencephalon with complete transection of lemniscal and indirect pain pathways in the reticular formation, and in the thalamus with destruction of thalamic nuclei do not threaten the patient with possible respiratory failure, they may, however, result in other serious disturbances as regards vegetative functions and affect consciousness and the psychic sphere too. Bilateral thalamotomy of the n.v.c.pc. in a single stage has so far been done only sporadically. ROWBOTHAM (1960) reports tenacious headache and facial pain following bilateral vascular affection of the centrum medianum and part of the n.v.c.

MONNIER used a two stage procedure for bilateral thalamotomy and observed the emergence of thalamic syndrome as a sequel. COOPER (1965) in two of his four cases operated for phantom pain achieved success only after thalamotomy performed in the second stage on the contralateral side. In the first patient he performed destruction of the ventrooral nucleus for parkinsonism, and simultaneously destruction of n.v.c. for phantom pain on the left side. After one year, during right thalamotomy n.v.o. he did simultaneously destruction of n.v.c. on the same side, as the patient complained of return of phantom pain soon after the first operation. Complete disappearance of pain resulted from the second operation. Based on this experience, COOPER, in a second patient with phantom pain, performed contralateral thalamotomy already 8 days after the first intervention. Symptoms were completely relieved, despite the fact that the patient had already got used to high doses of opiates. COOPER, in this connection, emphasizes the importance of destruction of pathways that do not cross over for influencing central pain. If later results should confirm the accuracy of COOPER's observations, bilateral operation would bring about substantial progress in controlling intractable central pain.

More frequent reports have been published on cases submitted to destruction of the dorsomedial thalamic nucleus on one side and to destruction of n.v.c. or mesencephalotomy on the other. The writer performed five bilateral mesencephalic tractotomies, segmental without exception, complete dissection, also including the reticular formation, was never performed. However, also these operations done in a single stage, were associated with prolonged recovery of consciousness, as if the operation had been done under a general anaesthetic, as well as with shortlived psychological upsets, or temporary confusion. Bearing in mind all these possible complications, we decided to perform in cases with bilateral pain, operations in the mesencephalon or thalamus on one side, and upper thoracic chordotomy on the other (Tables 3 and 4). Both interventions are done in one session, in the sitting position. A disadvantage of this is the great loss of cerebrospinal fluid with accumulation of air in the ventricles and subarachnoidal spaces accompanied by headache during operation and persisting for several days. Results with these combined operations are otherwise excellent, pain in the midline is completely relieved as is visceral pain.

Where pain is associated with a marked emotional component, some authors perform partial destruction of the n. dorsomedialis thalami. They restrict operation in some cases to this procedure, in others they combine it with mesencephalic tractotomy, or destruction of the n.v.c.pc. in the thalamus. The writer endeavours to achieve the same object, i.e. modify the psychological element, by transection of frontothalamic tracts on the border between lateral and medial thalamic nuclear structures by the so-called partial longitudinal thalamotomy.

8. The Advantages and the Future of Thalamic Destructions

Unilateral destruction of the n.v.c.pc. with the neighbouring intrathalamic nuclei and with the subthalamic region does not as a rule produce major neurological defects. Temporary cerebellar disturbances may arise, which means that the cerebellodentato-rubrothalamic tract terminating in the n.v.i. (VL) has been affected. Sometimes also temporary motor disturbances due to a capsular lesion develop. The mortality of thalamotomy in the writer's series is 13.6%.

Neither has thalamotomy, despite the advantages described, so far been applied widely. This is not only caused by the fact that this method is much more recent than e.g. chordotomy, but mainly because it is a more complicated operation attacking an important area of the brain stem and, if stereotaxis is used, also much more expensive.

The writer, based on personal experience, has come to the conclusion that the opportunity of using an open approach within a distance of only a few millimetres from the desired structures and their destruction under visual control have greatly simplified the antalgic operations on the stem. As regards inconvenience caused to the patient and surgical risk they may be compared with chordotomy. The site of destruction in open thalamotomy is fixed and stable, thus the need for control by stimulation may be dispensed with if the loop scalpel is used, particularly if we bear in mind that it is desirable to destroy also the neighbouring nuclei in order to obtain a permanent effect. Such an intervention fulfills, therefore, perfectly, the demands made by HASSLER and RIECHERT (1959) i.e. that operation in the thalamus for intractable pain must be particularly accurate, more accurate than pallidotomy for extrapyramidal diseases.

Thalamotomy represents an important advance in the treatment of intractable pain. New knowledge on the optimal extent of destructions necessary in a sufficiently large area will be gained by growing experiences. The effect of operation is enhanced, whereas undesirable defects are getting less and are transitory as a rule. The open operation itself, lasting only 45—60 minutes causes no great inconvenience to the patient.

In the writer's opinion thalamotomy possesses the greatest number of advantages amongst all surgical procedures on the brain stem mentioned. Its risk is not too great, secondary defects are only transitory and not particularly significant and its effect is most hopeful. In contrast to mesencephalotomy, its great advantage lies in the fact that troublesome hyperpathias are much less frequent. Destruction of the n.v.c.pc. and some intrathalamic nuclei may in addition be combined with partial destruction of frontothalamic fibres, particularly in cases with a prominent psychic component, or in the presence of central pains. For the above-mentioned reasons thalamotomy for intractable pain is recommended on a growing scale.

VII. Conclusion

A historical review of operations in the region of the mesencephalon and thalamus reveals convincingly how great the difficulties were that arose and how many various obstacles had to be overcome, in order to devise a safe approach to these structures and to avoid serious and undesirable neurological defects originating from these interventions.

The region of the midbrain and thalamus drew an ever increasing attention also in connection with radical therapy of intractable pain, mainly if located in the upper parts of the body and of visceral or central pains. It is well known that the morphology of tracts conducting painful stimuli is getting increasingly complicated in the region of the midbrain and thalamus, accordingly interventions there are more exacting from all aspects. On the other hand these pathways are sufficiently distant from the respiratory centres at these levels, which means that complications directly endangering the patient's life need no longer be feared in association with their unilateral destruction.

The frequent emergence of postoperative hyperpathias and impairment of hearing played a major part in retarding the wider application of mesencephalotomy. Operations in the midbrain were for this reason modified and destruction of pathways made on the borderline between mesencephalon and thalamus. The incidence of both complications was reduced by selecting this site.

Open operations using the occipital supra-transtentorial approach of WALKER have been abandoned in due course and stereotaxis is used instead. This method facilitates intervention at the junction of mesencephalon and thalamus, as well as directly in the thalamic nuclei, up to that time inaccessible by the open route.

The present writer, during the years 1954—1956, devised an open infratentorial surgical approach creating relatively easy access to the midbrain, as well as to all parts of the thalamus and subthalamus in which surgeons are interested for the relief of pain; a total of 70 operations in 51 patients were done by the writer using this method. During the first phase, the years 1955—1957, operations performed consisted mainly of mesencephalic tractotomies, many of them segmental, and bilateral operations. During the next period,

1958—1960, pain pathways were transected at a somewhat higher
level, at the junction of mesencephalon and thalamus, in the so-
called porta thalami. At present, destruction of pain pathways is
done as they terminate in the thalamic nuclei, also by the open
infratentorial approach, after stereotactic operations for intractable
pain performed by various writers showed promising results.

Destruction in the mesencephalon and at the mesencephalothalamic junction is done with a curved scalpel with one-sided cutting
edge, destruction in the thalamus by a specially constructed probe,
armed with a retractable loop. The open infratentorial approach
associated with direct visualization of the posterior thalamic region
offers the great advantage of facilitating transection not only of
the closely adjoining parvocellular portion of the ventrocaudal
nucleus with the terminus of the specific pain pathway, but also
the major portion of the truncothalamic system, where the secondary pain pathways terminate or pass through. This may be achieved
by stereotaxis only at the price of more extensive, undesirable destruction of other sections of the thalamus, particularly those located dorsally.

In central pain, or in cases with a prominent emotional reaction
of the patient against severe organic pain, some writers perform
also destruction of the medial thalamic nucleus. Experiences revealed that this operation, even if done on only one side and fairly
extensively, may result in as grave personality defects as are a
regular sequel of bilateral frontal lobotomy. The writer substituted
for this step the transection of only a limited portion of frontothalamic pathways at the junction of lateral and medial groups of
thalamic nuclear structures. This is designated "partial longitudinal
thalamotomy."

Amongst all the interventions that may at present be applied
for treating intractable pain in the upper parts of the body, in pain
situated in the midline, in diffusely located visceral pains or finally
in central pain, thalamotomy appears to hold out the greatest
promise of success at present. To render destruction in the thalamus
more accurate by using the open approach route and make this
method as safe and as effective as possible, were in brief the objects
of the writer's endeavour. The open approach, though not simpler
than stereotaxis, nevertheless has the advantage of being performed
under direct visual control, rendering it more accurate, decidedly
less timeconsuming and easier, in particular for anybody making
themselves well acquainted with the technique of this operation and
the topography of the posterior incisural region.

References

ADAMS, J. E., and D. MUNRO: Cited by BIRKENFELD, R., and R. G. FISHER, in: J. Neurosurg. **20**, 303—311 (1963).

BAGGENSTOSS, A. H., and J. G. LOVE: Pinealomas. Arch. Neurol. Psychiat. **41**, 1187—1206 (1939).

BAILEY, P., and E. W. DAVIS: Effects of lesions of the periaqueductal gray matter of Macaca mulatta. J. Neuropath. **3**, 69—72 (1944).

BAILEY, R. A., P. GLEES, and D. R. OPPENHEIMER: Midbrain tractotomy. Mschr. Psychiat. Neurol. **127**, 316—335 (1954).

LE BEAU, J.: Anterior cingulectomy. J. Neurosurg. **11**, 268—276 (1954).

BECHTĚREW, W. v.: Über die Schleifenschicht auf Grund der Resultate von nach der entwicklungsgeschichtlichen Methode ausgeführten Untersuchungen. Arch. Anat. Entw.gesch., Leipzig, 1895, 379. Cited by R. HASSLER, in: Acta Neurochirurg. **8**, 353—423 (1960).

BELMUSTO, L., E. BROWN, and G. OWENS: Clinical observations on respiration and vasomotor disturbance as related to cervical cordotomies. J. Neurosurg. **20**, 225—232 (1963).

BETTAG, W., and T. YOSHIDA: Über stereotaktische Schmerzoperationen. Acta Neurochirurg. **8**, 299—317 (1960).

BIRKENFELD, R., and R. G. FISHER: Successful treatment of causalgia of upper extremity with medullary spinothalamic tractotomy. J. Neurosurg. **20**, 303—311 (1963).

BLOMQUIST, A. J., R. M. BENJAMIN, and R. EMMERS: Thalamic localization of afferents from the tongue in squirrel monkey. J. Compar. Neurol. **118**, 77—81 (1962).

BOHM, E.: Chordotomy for intractable pain due to malignant disease. Acta Psychiat. Neurol. Scand. **35**, 145—155 (1960).

BOWSHER, D.: Termination of the central pain pathway in man. Brain **80**, 606 —622 (1957).

— The reticular formation and ascending reticular system: anatomical considerations. Brit. J. Anaesth. **33**, 174—182 (1961).

BRODAL, A.: The reticular formation of the brain stem. Edinburgh: Oliver and Boyd. 1957.

— F. WALBERG, and T. BLACKSTAD: Termination of spinal afferents to inferior olive in cat. J. Neurophysiol. **13**, 341—454 (1950).

BRUNNER, C.: Zur Pathologie und Operabilität der Tumoren der Zirbeldrüse. Beitr. z. klin. Chir. **83**, 451—474 (1913). Cited by E. WALKER, in: A history of neurological surgery. Baltimore: The Williams & Wilkins Co. 1951.

BUCY, P. C., J. E. KEPLINGER, and E. B. SIQUEIRA: Destruction of the "pyramidal tract" in man. J. Neurosurg. **21**, 385—398 (1964).

CHANG, H. T., and T. C. RUCH: Topographical distribution of spinothalamic fibres in the thalamus of the spider monkey. J. Anat. **81**, 150—164 (1947).

CLARK, W. E., and LE GROS: The structure and connections of the thalamus. Brain 55, 406—470 (1932).

— — The termination of ascending tracts in the thalamus of the Macaque monkey. J. Anat. 71, 7—40 (1936).

CONSTANS, J. P.: Chirurgie frontale de la douleur. Acta Neurochirurg. 8, 251—281 (1960).

COOPER, I. S.: Intracerebral injection of procain into the globus pallidus in hyperkinetic disorders. Science 119, 417—418 (1954).

— The neurosurgical alleviation of parkinsonism. Springfield, Ill.: Ch. C. Thomas. 1956.

— Clinical and physiological implications of thalamic surgery for disorders of sensory communication. Part 1. Thalamic surgery for intractable pain. J. Neurol. Sci. 2, 493—519 (1965).

CRAWFORD, A. S.: Medullary tractotomy for relief of intractable pain in upper levels. Arch. Surg. 55, 523—529 (1947).

— Medullary spinothalamic tractotomy for high intractable pain. J. Maine med. Ass. 51, 233—235 (1960).

— and R. S. KNIGHTON: Further observations on medullary spinothalamic tractotomy. J. Neurosurg. 10, 113—121 (1953).

DANDY, W. E.: An operation for the removal of pineal tumors. Surg. Gynec. Obst. 33, 113—119 (1921).

DAVID, M., J. TALAIRACH, and H. HÉCAEN: Etude critique des interventions neurochirurgicales actuellement pratiqués dans le traitement de la douleur. Sem. Hôp., Paris 23, 1651—1665 (1947).

DÉJÉRINE, J., and G. ROUSSY: Le syndrome thalamique. Rev. Neurol. 14, 521—532 (1906).

DOGLIOTTI, M.: First surgical section in man of the lemniscus lateralis. Curr. Res. Anaest. Analg. 17, 143—145 (1938).

DRAKE, C. G., and K. G. McKENZIE: Mesencephalic tractotomy for pain. J. Neurosurg. 10, 457—462 (1953).

FALCONER, M. A.: Intramedullary trigeminal tractotomy and its place in the treatment of facial pain. J. Neurol. Neurosurg. Psychiat. 12, 297—311 (1949).

FÖRSTER, O.: Die Leitungsbahnen des Schmerzgefühls. Wien: Urban & Schwarzenberg. 1927.

— Das operative Vorgehen bei Tumoren der Vierhügelgegend. Wien. klin. Wschr. 41, 986—990 (1928).

— and O. GAGEL: Die Vorderseitenstrangdurchschneidung beim Menschen. Z. ges. Neurol. Psychiat. 138, 1—92 (1932).

FOLTZ, E. L., and L. E. WHITE, JR.: Pain "relief" by frontal cingulotomy. J. Neurosurg. 19, 89—100 (1962).

FREEMAN, W., and J. W. WATTS: Prefrontal lobotomy in agitated depression. Report of a case. M. Ann. District of Columbia 5, 326—328 (1936). Cited by E. WALKER, in: A history of neurological surgery. Baltimore: The Williams & Wilkins Co. 1951.

— — Pain of organic disease relieved by prefrontal lobotomy. Lancet 250, 953—955 (1946).

FRENCH, L. A., G. L. HAINES, and W. S. OGLE: Differential section of the spinothalamic tract to relieve pain from carcinoma of the breast. Surgery 39, 107—113 (1956).

FRY, W.J., R. MEYERS, D. F. SCHULTZ, L. L. DREYER, and R. F. NOYES: Topical differentia of pathogenetic mechanisms underlying Parkinsonian tremor and rigidity as indicated by ultrasonic irradiation of the human brain. Transactions Amer. Neurol. Ass. 1958, 18—24.

FUSEK, I., and L. PAVLÍČEK: Kryosonda pro stereotaktickou neurochirurgii. Rozhl. chir. 43, 689—692 (1964).

GARDNER, E. D., and F. MORIN: Spinal pathways for projection of cutaneous and muscular afferents to the sensory and motor cortex of the monkey. Amer. J. Physiol. 174, 149—154 (1953).

GLEES, P.: The central pain tract. Acta Neuroveget. 7, 160—174 (1953).

— and R. A. BAILEY: Schichtung und Fasergröße des Tractus spinothalamicus des Menschen. Mschr. Psychiat. Neurol. 122, 129—141 (1951).

GRANT, F. C., and F. A. WOOD: Experiences with cordotomy. Clin. Neurosurg. 5, 38—64 (1958).

GRANTHAM, E. G.: Prefrontal lobotomy for relief of pain, with a report of a new operative technique. J. Neurosurg. 8, 405—410 (1951).

GUIOT, G., and S. FORJAZ: La tractotomie mésencéphalique par voie sous-temporale. Rev. Neurol. 79, 733—740 (1947).

HASSLER, R.: Die Anatomie des Thalamus. Arch. Psychiat. 184, 249—256 (1950).
— Anatomie des Thalamus. G. SCHALTENBRAND and P. BAILEY: Introduction to stereotaxis with an atlas of the human brain, pp. 230—290. Stuttgart: G. Thieme. 1959.
— and T. RIECHERT: Indikationen und Lokalisationsmethode der gezielten Hirnoperationen. Nervenarzt 25, 441—447 (1954).
— — Klinische und anatomische Befunde bei stereotaktischen Schmerzoperationen im Thalamus. Arch. Psychiat. Nervenkr. 200, 93—122 (1959).

HEAD, H., W. H. R. RIVERS, and J. SHERREN: The afferent nervous system from a new aspect. Brain 28, 99—115 (1905).
— and G. HOLMES: Sensory disturbances from cerebral lesions. Brain 34, 102—254 (1912).

HORRAX, G.: Extirpation of a huge pinealoma from a patient with pubertas praecox. Arch. Neurol. Psychiat. 37, 385—397 (1937).
— and J. T. DANIELS: The conservative treatment of pineal tumors. Surg. Clin. North Amer. 22, 649—659 (1942).
— and W. T. PRICE, JR.: High cervical chordotomy for relief of intractable pain in the arm, shoulder and upper chest. Ann. Surg. 139, 567—585 (1954).

HORSLEY, V., and R. H. CLARKE: The structure and functions of the cerebellum by a new method. Brain 31, 45—124 (1908).
— Discussion of paper by C. M. H. HOWELL, on tumors of the pineal body. Proc. Roy. Soc. Med. 3 (pt. 2) (neurol. section): 77. Cited by E. WALKER, in: A history of neurological surgery, p. 138. Baltimore: The Williams & Wilkins Co. 1951.

HUNSPERGER, R. W.: Affektreaktionen auf elektrische Reizung im Hirnstamm der Katze. Helvet. Physiol. Pharmacol. Acta 14, 70—92 (1956).

KAHN, E. A., and R. W. RAND: On the anatomy of anterolateral cordotomy. J. Neurosurg. 9, 611—619 (1952).

KARPLUS, J. P., and A. KREIDL: Gehirn und Sympathicus. 2. Mitteilung. Ein Sympathicuszentrum im Zwischenhirn. Arch. Physiol. norm. path. 135, 401—416 (1910). Cited by F. ROEDER and H. ORTHNER, in: Erfahrungen mit stereotaktischen Eingriffen, III. Mitteilung: Conf. Neurol. 21, 51—97 (1961).

KNIGHTON, R. S.: Thalamic relay nucleus for the second somatic sensory receiving area in the cerebral cortex of the cat. J. Comp. Neurol. **92**, 183—191 (1950).

KRAUSE, F.: Operative Freilegung der Vierhügel nebst Beobachtungen über Hirndruck und Dekompression. Zentralbl. Chir. **53**, 2812—2819 (1926).

KRUGEL, L.: Characteristics of somatic afferent projection to precentral cortex in monkey. Amer. J. Physiol. **186**, 475—482 (1956).

KUNC, Z.: Vztah aferentních vláken n. facialis, glossopharyngicus a vagus k tractus spinalis n. trigemini. Čs. neurol. **20**, 225—232 (1957).

— La localisation des trajets de la douleur des nerfs IX, X et VII dans la mœlle allongée et la possibilité de leur tractotomie sélective. Acta Neurochir. **8**, 327 to 334 (1960).

— and J. ŠIMEK: Neuralgie n. glossopharyngici vyléčená tractotomií podle Sjöqvista. Neurol. psychiatr. čsl. **18**, 135—137 (1955).

— and J. MARŠALA: La localisation et la terminaison des voies afferentes des nerfs IX et X dans le bulbe. Acta Neurochir. **10**, 512—522 (1962).

KURU, M.: Sensory path in the spinal cord and brain stem of man. Tokyo and Osaka: Sogensya, 1949, 39 pp. Cited by L. C. WHITE and W. H. SWEET, in: Pain. Springfield, Ill.: Ch. C. Thomas. 1955.

LANDAU, W., and G. H. BISHOP: Pain from dermal, periosteal and fascial endings and from inflammation. Arch. Neurol. Psychiat. **69**, 490—504 (1953).

LANDGREN, S.: Cortical reception of cold impulses from the tongue of the cat. Acta Physiol. Scand. **40**, 202—209 (1957).

— Convergence of tactile, thermal and gustatory impulses on single cortical cells. Acta Physiol. Scand. **40**, 210—221 (1957).

LEKSELL, L.: Gezielte Hirnoperationen. Handbuch Neurochirurgie **6**, 178—218 (1957).

LIVINGSTON, W. K.: Pain Mechanisms: A physiologic interpretation of causalgia and its related states. New York: Macmillan. 1943.

MARK, V. H., F. R. ERVIN, and T. P. HACKETT: Clinical aspects of stereotactic thalamotomy in the human. Part I. The treatment of chronic severe pain. Arch. Neurol. **3**, 351—367 (1960).

— — and P. I. YAKOVLEV: Stereotactic thalamotomy: III. Verification of anatomical lesion sites in human thalamus. Arch. Neurol. **8**, 528—538 (1963).

MASSETTI, F.: Dell'operabilità a delle vie di acceso ai tumori della ghiandola pineale. Policlin. Roma **20**, 497—501 (1913). Cited by E. WALKER, in: A history of neurological surgery. Baltimore: The Williams & Wilkins Co. 1951.

MAZARS, G., A. PANSINI, and J. CHIARELLI: Coagulation du faisceau spinothalamique et du faisceau quintothalamique par stéréotaxie. Rev. Neurol. **100**, 516 (1959).

— R. ROGE, and A. PANSINI: Stereotactic coagulation of the spinothalamic tract for intractable trigeminal pain. J. Neurol. Neurosurg. Psychiat. **23**, 352 (1960).

McKINLEY, W. A., and H. W. MAGOUN: The termination of ascending trigeminal and spinal tracts in the thalamus of the cat. Amer. J. Physiol. **137**, 409—416 (1942).

MEHLER, W. R.: The mammalian "pain tract" in phylogeny. Anat. Rec. **127**, 332 (1957).

— M. E. FEFERMAN, and W. J. H. NAUTA: Ascending axon degeneration following anterolateral chordotomy in the monkey. Anat. Rec. **124**, 332—333 (1956).

MEYERS, R., W. J. FRY, F. J. FRY, L. L. DREYER, D. F. SCHULTZ, and R. F. NOYES: Early experiences with ultrasonic irradiation of the pallidofugal and nigral complexes in hyperkinetic and hypertonic disorders. J. Neurosurg. 16, 32—54 (1959).

MIKULA, F., J. ŠIROKÝ, and B. ZAPLETAL: Le traitement des crises gastriques par la tractotomie mésencéphalique bilaterale et ses complications auditives inattendues. Rev. Oto-Neuro-Ophthal. 31, 1—8 (1959).

MONNIER, M.: Repérage, stimulation et coagulation thérapeutique des centres sous corticaux chez le singe et l'homme. Schweiz. Arch. Neurol. Psychiat. 67, 217 à 221 (1951).

— Les résultats de la coagulation du thalamus chez l'homme. (Noyau vetropostérieur.) Acta neurochir. Suppl. 3, 281—307 (1955).

MORIN, F., H. G. SCHWARZ, and J. L. LEARY: Experimental study of the spinothalamic and related tracts. Acta Psychiat. Scand. 26, 371—396 (1951).

MORUZZI, G., and H. W. MAGOUN: Brain stem reticular formation and activation of the EEG. EEG Clin. Neurophysiol. 1, 454—473 (1949).

MOUNTCASTLE, V. B., and E. HENNEMAN: The representation of tactile sensibility in the thalamus of the monkey. J. Comp. Neurol. 97, 409—440 (1952).

NOORDENBOS, W.: Einige theoretische Bemerkungen über den zentralen Schmerz. Acta Neurochir. 8, 113—120 (1959).

OBRADOR, S.: A simplified neurosurgical technique for approaching and damaging the region of the globus pallidus in Parkinson's disease. J. Neurol. Neurosurg. Psychiat. 20, 47—49 (1957).

OGLE, W. S., L. A. FRENCH, and W. T. PEYTON: Experiences with high cervical chordotomy. J. Neurosurg. 13, 81—87 (1956).

OPPENHEIMER, H., and F. KRAUSE: Operative Erfolge bei Geschwülsten der Sehhügel und Vierhügelgegend. Berl. klin. Wschr. 50, 2316—2322 (1913).

ORTHNER, H.: Pathologische Anatomie der vom Hypothalamus ausgelösten Bewußtseinsstörungen. I. Internat. Kongr. Neurol. Wiss. 2, 77—96 (1957).

PATTON, H. D., T. C. RUCH, and A. E. WALKER: Experimental hypogeusia from horsley-clarke lesions of the thalamus in Macaca Mulatta. J. Neurophysiol. 7, 171—184 (1944).

PAVLONSKIJ, A. M., and K. I. PENKOVOJ: Operativnye postupy k opucholjam golovnogo mozga, prochodjaščim čerez tentorialnoe otverstie. Vop. Nějrochir. 1962, 24—27.

PETRÉN, K.: Über die Bahnen der Sensibilität im Rückenmarke, besonders nach den Fällen von Stichverletzung studiert. Arch. Psychiat. 47, 495—557 (1910).

POWELL, T. P. S., and W. M. COWAN: A study of thalamus-striate relations in the monkey. Brain 79, 364—381 (1956).

PUUSEPP, L.: Die operative Entfernung einer Zyste der glandula pinealis. Neurol. Centralbl. 33, 560—563 (1914). Cited by E. WALKER, in: A history of neurological surgery. Baltimore: The Williams & Wilkins Co. 1951.

RAND, C. T., W. F. COLLINS, H. S. DAVIS, and W. H. DILLON: Differential susceptibility of afferent pathways to anesthetic agents in the cat. Amer. J. Physiol. 192, 305—310 (1958).

RAND, R. W.: Substantia nigralysis. A new surgical technique for treatment of Parkinson's disease and other hyperkinetic syndromes. Bull. Los Angeles Neurol. Soc. 24, 214—216 (1959).

RANSON, S. W., and H. W. MAGOUN: The central path of the pupilloconstrictor reflex in response to light. Arch. Neurol. Psychiat. **30**, 1193—1202 (1933).

RIECHERT, T.: Die stereotaktischen Hirnoperationen in ihrer Anwendung bei den Hyperkinesen, bei Schmerzzuständen und einigen weiteren Indikationen. I. Internat. Kongr. Neurochir., Acta med. belg., Bruxelles **1957**, 121—160.

— Über die Technik und einige Indikationen der gezielten Hirnoperationen. Nervenarzt **30**, 385—391 (1959).

— Die chirurgische Behandlung der zentralen Schmerzzustände einschließlich der stereotaktischen Operationen im Thalamus und Mesencephalon. Acta Neurochir. **8**, 136—152 (1960).

— and F. MUNDINGER: Beschreibung und Anwendung eines Zielgerätes für stereotaktische Hirnoperationen. Acta Neurochir. Suppl. **3**, 308—337 (1956).

— and R. SCHWARZ: Erfahrungen mit kortikalen und intrazerebralen Ableitungen der Hirnströme. Dtsch. med. Wschr. **77**, 1075—1077 (1952).

— and M. WOLF: Ein neues Zielgerät für die Koagulation des Ganglion Gasseri und andere intrazerebrale Eingriffe. Acta Neurochir. **2**, 27—28 (1952).

ROEDER, F., and H. ORTHNER: Erfahrungen mit stereotaktischen Eingriffen. III. Mitteilung. Confin. Neurol. **21**, 51—97 (1961).

ROWBOTHAM, G. F.: A case of intractable pain in the head and face associated with pathological changes in the optic thalamus. Acta Neurochir. **9**, 1—8 (1960).

SCARFF, J. E.: Unilateral prefrontal lobotomy for the relief of intractable pain. Report of 58 cases with special consideration of failures. J. Neurosurg. **7**, 330—336 (1950).

SCHALTENBRAND, G., and P. BAILEY: Einführung in die stereotaktischen Operationen mit einem Atlas des menschlichen Gehirns, Band I—III. Stuttgart: G. Thieme. 1959.

SCHWARTZ, H. G., and J. L. O'LEARY: Section of the spinothalamic tract in the medulla with observations on the pathway for pain. Surgery **9**, 183—193 (1941).

— — Section of the spinothalamic tract at the level of the inferior olive. Arch. Neurol. Psychiat. **47**, 293—304 (1942).

SJÖQVIST, O.: Eine neue Operationsmethode bei Trigeminusneuralgie: Durchschneidung des Tractus spinalis trigemini. Zbl. Neurochir. **2**, 274—281 (1937).

SPIEGEL, E. A., H. T. WYCIS, M. MARKS, and A. J. LEE: Stereotaxic apparatus for operations on human brain. Science **106**, 349—350 (1947).

— — Principles et applications de la stéréoencéphalotomie. Acta Neurochir. **1**, 137—153 (1950).

— — and H. FREED: Stereoencephalotomy. Thalamotomy and related procedures. J. A. M. A. **148**, 446—451 (1952).

— — Mesencephalotomy in treatment of "intractable" facial pain. Arch. Neurol. Psychiat. **69**, 1—13 (1953).

— M. KLEIZKIN, E. G. SZEKELY, and H. T. WYCIS: Role of hypothalamic mechanisms in thalamic pain. Neurology **4**, 739—751 (1954).

SPILLER, W. G., and E. MARTIN: The treatment of persistent pain of organic origin in the lower part of the body by division of the anterolateral column of the spinal cord. J. A. M. A. **58**, 1489—1490 (1912).

SPIVY, D. F., and J. S. METCALF: Differential effect of medial and lateral dorsal root sections upon subcortical evoked potentials. J. Neurophysiol. **22**, 367—373 (1959).

STOPFORD, J. S. B.: The function of the spinal nucleus of the trigeminal nerve. J. Anat. **59**, 120—728 (1925).

SWEET, W. H., V. H. MARK, and H. HAMLIN: Radiofrequency lesions in the central nervous system of man and cat, including case reports of eight bulbar pain-tract interruptions. J. Neurosurg. **17**, 213—225 (1960).

TALAIRACH, J.: Chirurgie stéréotaxique du thalamus. VI. Congrès Latinoamer. Neurochir., Montevideo, 1955, pp. 865—925.

— H. HÉCAEN, M. DAVID, M. MONNIER, and J. AJURIAGUERRA: Recherches sur la coagulation thérapeutique des structures sous-corticales chez l'homme. Rev. Neurol. **81**, 4—24 (1949).

TANDLER, J., and E. RANZI: Chirurgische Anatomie und Operationstechnik des Zentralnervensystems. Berlin: J. Springer. 1920. Cited by E. WALKER, in: A history of neurological surgery. Baltimore: The Williams & Wilkins Co. 1951.

TORVIK, A.: Sensory, motor and reflex changes in two cases of intractable pain after stereotactic mesencephalic tractotomy. J. Neurol. Neurosurg. Psychiat. **22**, 299—305 (1959).

— and A. BRODAL: The origin of reticulospinal fibres in the cat. An experimental study. Anat. Record. **128**, 113—118 (1957).

UMBACH, W.: Elektrophysiologische und vegetative Phänomene bei stereotaktischen Hirnoperationen. Berlin-Heidelberg-New York: Springer. 1966.

VALVERDE, F.: Reticular formation of the pons and medulla oblongata. A Golgi study. J. Compar. Neurol. **116**, 71—99 (1961).

VOGT, C., and O. VOGT: Thalamusstudien I—III. J. Psychol. **50**, 32—154 (1941).

VAN WAGENEN, W. P.: A surgical approach for the removal of certain pineal tumors. Report of a case. Surg. Gynec. Obst. **53**, 216—220 (1931).

WALKER, A. E.: The primate thalamus. University of Chicago Press, 1938.

— The spinothalamic tract in man. Arch. Neurol. Psychiat. **43**, 284—298 (1940).

— Mesencephalic tractotomy. A method for relief of unilateral intractable pain. Arch. Surg. **44**, 953—962 (1942).

— Relief of pain by mesencephalic tractotomy. Arch. Neurol. Psychiat. **48**, 865—883 (1942).

— Somatotopic localization of spinothalamic and secondary trigeminal tracts in mesencephalon. Arch. Neurol. Psychiat. **48**, 884—889 (1942).

— Cerebral pedunculotomy for the relief of involuntary movements. I. Hemiballismus. Acta Psychiat. Neurol. **24**, 723—729 (1949).

— A history of neurological surgery. Baltimore: The Williams & Wilkins Co. 1951.

WALLENBERG, A: Die sekundäre Bahn des sensiblen Trigeminus. Anat. Anz. **12**, 95 110 (1896).

— Sekundäre sensible Bahnen im Gehirnstamme des Kaninchens, ihre gegenseitige Lage und ihre Bedeutung für den Aufbau des Thalamus. Anat. Anz. **18**, 81 (1900). Cited by R. HASSLER, in: Anatomie des Thalamus, 1959.

WATTS, J. W., and J. P. MURPHY: Psychosurgery: Surgical aspects. Chap. 21 B, in: Progress in Neurology and Psychiatry, pp. 395—401 (ed. E. A. SPIEGEL). New York: Grune & Stratton. 1949.

WEDDELL, G., D. C. SINCLAIR, and W. H. FEINDEL: An anatomical basis for alteration in quality of pain sensibility. J. Neurophysiol. **11**, 99—109 (1948).

WHITE, J. C.: Spinothalamic tractotomy in the medulla oblongata. An operation for the relief of intractable neuralgias of the occiput, neck and shoulder. Arch. Surg. **43**, 113—127 (1941).

— Modifications of frontal leukotomy for relief of pain and suffering in terminal malignant disease. Ann. Surg. **156,** 394—403 (1962).

WHITE, J. C., and W. H. SWEET: Pain. Its Mechanisms and Neurosurgical Control. Springfield, Ill.: Ch. C. Thomas. 1955.

WHITLOCK, D. G., and E. R. PERL: Afferent projections through ventrolateral funiculi to thalamus of cat. J. Neurophysiol. **22**, 113—148 (1959).

WYCIS, H. T., and E. A. SPIEGEL: Symposium: Psychosurgery. Thalamotomy and mesencephalotomy. Neurosurgical aspects (including treatment of pain). New York J. Med. **49**, 2275 (1949).

— L. SOLOFF, and E. A. SPIEGEL: Facial pain, persisting after retrogasserian rhizotomy, relieved by mesencephalothalamotomy. Surgery **27**, 115—121 (1950).

— and E. A. SPIEGEL: Long-range results in the treatment of intractable pain by stereotaxic midbrain surgery. J. Neurosurg. **19**, 101—107 (1962).

ZAPLETAL, B.: Výhody infratentoriální přístupové cesty ke čtyřhrbolí středního mozku a další možnosti chirurgické léčby neztišitelné bolesti mesencefalickou traktotomií. Acta Univ. Olomuc. **7**, 95—107 (1955).

— Ein neuer operativer Zugang zum Gebiet der Incisura Tentorii. Zbl. Neurochir. **16**, 64—69 (1956).

— Die mesencephale Traktotomie von einem infratentorialen Operationszugang. Bilaterale Mesencephalotomie. Zbl. Neurochir. **16**, 154—165 (1956).

— Nigrotomy in treatment of extrapyramidal diseases. Acta Neurochir. **13**, 388—392 (1965).

Subject Index